Well-Being and Cultures

Cross-Cultural Advancements in Positive Psychology

Volume 3

The aim of the *Cross Cultural Advancements in Positive Psychology* book series is to spread a universal and culture-fair perspective on good life promotion. The series will advance a deeper understanding of the cross-cultural differences in well-being conceptualization. A deeper understanding can affect psychological theories, interventions and social policies in various domains, from health to education, from work to leisure. Books in the series will investigate such issues as enhanced mobility of people across nations, ethnic conflicts and the challenges faced by traditional communities due to the pervasive spreading of modernization trends. New instruments and models will be proposed to identify the crucial components of well-being in the process of acculturation. This series will also explore dimensions and components of happiness that are currently overlooked because happiness research is grounded in the Western tradition, and these dimensions do not belong to the Western cultural frame of mind and values.

For further volumes:
http://www.springer.com/series/8420

Hans Henrik Knoop • Antonella Delle Fave
Editors

Well-Being and Cultures

Perspectives from Positive Psychology

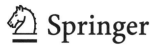 Springer

Editors
Hans Henrik Knoop
Department of Education
Aarhus University
Niels Juels Gade 84
8000 Aarhus, Denmark

Antonella Delle Fave
Dipartimento di Scienze Cliniche Luigi Sacco
Università degli Studi di Milano
Via G.B. Grassi 74
20157 Milano, Italy

ISSN 2210-5417   ISSN 2210-5425 (electronic)
ISBN 978-94-007-4610-7   ISBN 978-94-007-4611-4 (eBook)
DOI 10.1007/978-94-007-4611-4
Springer Dordrecht Heidelberg New York London

Library of Congress Control Number: 2012945199

Printed on acid-free paper

Springer is part of Springer Science+Business Media (www.springer.com)

Contents

Chapter 1
Positive Psychology and Cross-Cultural Research

Hans Henrik Knoop and Antonella Delle Fave

Prologue: One World, No Neighbours?

The 5th Biannual European Conference on Positive Psychology[1] conducted by the European Network for Positive Psychology (ENPP) was held in Copenhagen in June 2010. The conference was the largest in the history of the ENPP, and throughout 3 days the joy of cultural diversity was felt, if certainly in an atmosphere of shared appreciation and basic ethics. More than 300 submitted abstracts were accepted for presentation, focusing on a wide array of topics, many of which addressed cross-cultural issues of well-being and optimal functioning, and subsequently authors were invited to submit papers based on their presentations. This anthology represents an elaborated selection of these submissions offered to a broader readership.

Today, it is increasingly difficult to identify what exactly is meant by "cross-cultural", as the globalized world is merging to an extent that almost everything seems to transcend not only traditional geographical borders but also cultural ones, thus becoming multicultural almost by definition. Yet, in much of social science, the distinction between what is universal and cultural specific remains as important as ever, as multinational/international organizations sweep the globe, thereby in reality often bringing about a sort of "uni-culturality" that was not asked for in the first place. Cultural diversity is quintessential for human experience and for a colourful

---

[1] Conference website: www.enpp2010.dk

H.H. Knoop (✉)
Department of Education, Aarhus University, Aarhus, Denmark
e-mail: knoop@dpu.dk

A. Delle Fave
Dipartimento di Scienze Cliniche Luigi Sacco, Università degli Studi di Milano,
Milan, Italy
e-mail: antonella.dellefave@unimi.it

H.H. Knoop and A. Delle Fave (eds.), *Well-Being and Cultures: Perspectives from Positive Psychology*, Cross-Cultural Advancements in Positive Psychology 3, DOI 10.1007/978-94-007-4611-4_1, © Springer Science+Business Media Dordrecht 2013

global society, as humans quickly habituate to any given cultural setting, which thus soon loses its appeal if it does not continue to creatively develop its specialties. And as history shows, most new ideas come from others (i.e. Diamond 1997). So at a time where an airport in Thailand is barely distinguishable from one in Midwest United States or Northern Europe, with the same stores, offering the same products, expecting the same standards of behaviour, we know that we are not only privileged by this kind of "global harmony" but also threatened by a monolithic dominance behind this trend and widespread boredom in lack of neighbours. Certainly, the present ubiquitous social media and the increasing ability for many to travel do provide for new kinds of global neighbourhood, but even such fantastic improvements are bound to lose their appeal if cultural diversity collapses. At the very time of writing this chapter, a curious symptom of the aforementioned trend is the child celebrity, Justin Bieber, whose music video *Baby* records a mind-blowing 691,468,167 hits on the video sharing site YouTube – with 1,065,294 registered users "liking" it and more than twice as many, 2,203,747, who do not. If nothing else, this may serve as indication of how it is indeed possible to be very popular even though a majority does not like you.[2]

Individuals and Cultures: A Multifaceted Interaction

Several scholars have claimed that positive psychology shares with most other branches of the discipline an individualistic bias (Richardson and Guignon 2008). This bias consists in treating individuals as "fixed and essential selves", who autonomously shape their inner reality and their relationship with the environment (Christopher and Hickinbottom 2008), and it leads researchers to neglect the impact of cultural norms and beliefs on the subjective interpretation of happiness, well-being and quality of life (Becker and Marecek 2008). This problem, referred to as *conceptual individualism* (Kristjansson 2010), is not confined to positive psychology only; rather, it can be detected in most theories and interventions in psychology. Contextual factors are considered only to the extent that they are incorporated into the individual self-definitions, thus becoming isolated from the environment as components of stable and well-defined personal identities, in spite of the changes that both the environment and the individual ceaselessly undergo (Slife and Richardson 2008).

The issue of connecting positive psychology to social theories and paradigms has been systematically addressed prominently in studies on satisfaction with life and subjective well-being (Diener 2009; Veenhoven 2010); however, an increasing number of scientific publications are focusing on the cultural dimensions of other aspects of well-being. Nevertheless, a much more systematic work would be welcome, especially at the intervention level. While it is surely much easier to change

---

[2] Retrieved online, January 15, 2012, at: www.youtube.com/watch?v=kffacxfA7G4

individuals than institutions or social policies, paying attention to the individual/ environment interaction has proved to promote much more effective changes in the short as well as in the long run. A paradigmatic example of this broadening of perspectives comes from organizational psychology. While most studies on burnout and well-being promotion at work traditionally focused on individual intervention, aiming at reducing stress and improving coping strategies (Maslach and Goldberg 1998), more recent approaches also involve changes at the organizational, interpersonal and structural levels (Bakker et al. 2000; Gavin and Mason 2004; Maslach et al. 2001).

A related issue that has been only partially addressed by positive psychology, and that has great impact on methodological and analytical procedures, concerns the correspondence or equivalence of variables assessed at the cultural level or at the individual one. Several studies have highlighted the problem of isomorphism – or similarity of structures – between findings analyzed at the individual and cultural levels. The problem was raised two decades ago by Hofstede and his colleagues (1993) and has been receiving increasing attention, leading researchers to distinguish between culturally grounded and individually grounded variations in measures assessing various psychological constructs, ranging from cognitive variables to social orientations and emotions (Fischer 2009; Fischer et al. 2010; Kirkman et al. 2006; Na et al. 2010; Sauter et al. 2010).

Surely psychology, and in particular positive psychology, needs to develop stronger connections with other sciences such as sociology and economics (Oishi et al. 2009). However, from a more general point of view, studies involving culture have to deal with a substantial question concerning what comes first – the culture or the individual. This question can hardly get a unilateral answer, as the issue is extremely complex and calls into play the human ability for social learning.

The development of a cultural niche, in which individuals can acquire second-hand information from other members of their species, is a key factor in human fitness and adaptation, in that it allows individuals and groups to face daily challenges and to survive in a constantly changing environment (Richerson and Boyd 2005; Super and Harkness 1986; Strimling et al. 2009). In this complex system of information exchange, however, each person plays multiple roles, as heir, transformer and transmitter of cultural information (Acerbi et al. 2009; Laland et al. 2000; Boyd et al. 2011), in an interdependent process of circular causality with the cultural environment (Massimini and Delle Fave 2000).

This circularity process can be detected at any level of investigation. Decision-making forces are at work in human history, and they prevail on random changes: individual intentionality and direction are two crucial elements supporting cultural survival and transmission (Jablonka and Lamb 2005). Individual cognition directs social learning and makes use of the available cultural information according to principles that deeply differ from random selection, such as biases related to the information contents, the situations in which information is exchanged, and its popularity within the group (Henrich et al. 2008; Newson et al. 2007). Moreover, individuals are able to introduce innovations at both the material and conceptual levels at any time throughout the history of a society, by inventing new variants of objects and ideas, or by modifying previously existing ones (Delle Fave et al. 2011b). These variants are subsequently encoded in extrasomatic carriers through processes of externalization, anonymization, institutionalization and ritualization (Bateson and Hinde 1976). Humans used their ability for self-description to develop collective prescriptions, progressively moving from the micro-level of individuality and contingent interaction to the macro-level of groups and institutionalized relations (Berger and Luckman 1966). Within a social system, each person is connected to the cultural meanings through idiosyncratic processes of internalization and externalization (Vaalsiner 1998, 2007). Collective-cultural meanings are transformed into subjective reconstructions and can be externalized through individual behaviours, goals and strivings.

In the light of the circularity relationship between individual and culture, the recurrent finding that cultural differences and individual differences do not necessarily overlap should not be surprising. For example, recent studies in the well-being domain highlighted differences between cultural values and individual subjective concepts of good actions or good life, in terms of both their verbal definitions and their behavioural practice (Tafarodi et al. 2011). While values are characterized by a high degree of abstraction, people usually evaluate behaviours or situations according to more empirical and emotion-laden meanings and ideals (Leung and Bond 2004; Freeman and Brockmeier 2001). To address this crucial issue, it can be necessary to modify or split models and theoretical constructs: an exemplary case is Schwartz value theory, which comprises one model to evaluate individual differences and one to investigate cultural differences (Schwartz 1992, 2006). In addition, within the same society, contextual aspects, such as socio-economic status and education as well as historical changes, can affect individual evaluations (Inglehart and Baker 2000).

Researchers in positive psychology are increasingly paying attention to these topics. Cross-cultural comparisons have been conducted on various constructs through quantitative instruments and analyses (Diener et al. 2003; Park et al. 2006) as well as through qualitative studies and mixed-method approaches (Delle Fave and Bassi 2009; Delle Fave et al. 2011a, b; Lu and Gilmour 2006). Nevertheless, well-being is a topic universally addressed throughout history and across traditions and societies, and there is still wide place for exploration and understanding.

Composition of This Volume

In line with the premises outlined in the previous section, this anthology maintains a specific approach, as all the authors focus on *empirical studies comparing cultures* as concerns important positive psychological topics. As editors of this volume, we are not implying, let alone investigating in any detail, whether global economic and social trends are overall good, socially justified, done on purpose or brought about by sheer emergence of unpredictable market forces. Our aim is much more humble. We simply wish to contribute to a broader understanding of positive psychology between and across cultures by providing a medium for highly talented and concerned researchers working on important issues of human living. And we trust to have done so.

The volume includes 12 contributions. The first two chapters focus on theoretical approaches and instruments developed to assess happiness and well-being across cultures. First, Ryan Niemiec is offering a first-hand overview of the first decade with the Values in Action (VIA) Classification of Strengths (Peterson and Seligman 2004). In his chapter, Niemiec shows how the VIA Classification is now a recognized framework for helping individuals discover, explore and use their character strengths. Likewise, the derived VIA Inventory of Strengths is widely used as an assessment instrument that measures 24 universally valued strengths. Niemiec shares insights into important links between these character strengths and valued outcomes like life satisfaction and achievement, along with considerations regarding promising and potential further applications.

In the second chapter, Carmelo Vázquez and Gonzalo Hervas introduce the Pemberton Happiness Index, a new instrument for measuring well-being across cultures. This instrument is a brief measure of integrative well-being that taps into general, hedonic, eudaemonic, and social well-being, and that combines two methodologies to comprise both remembered and experienced well-being. Moving from a discussion on the multifaceted problems concerning the definition and assessment of well-being, the authors describe how the Pemberton Happiness Index represents an effort to overcome these problems. Specific attention is given to what and how to measure, as well as how to do this time and cost efficiently.

The following five chapters address the relationship between well-being, cultures and values. The first contribution, by Hilde Eileen Nafstad, Rolv Mikkel Blakar, Albert Botchway, Erlend Sand Bruer, Petra Filkukova and Kim Rand-Hendriksen, offers a conception of globalization as an ideology or worldview that is, as a system of ideas and values, circulating in the public realm and influencing societies worldwide, thereby defining and articulating local values and visions for social change. The authors analyze the influences of globalization on communal values and sense of community as reflected in the language used in public discourses (newspapers) in three different societies: a post-communist East European republic (The Czech Republic), a Nordic welfare state (Norway), and a modern West African society (Ghana).

Following, Ognen Spasovski explores the perception of subjective well-being in a post-communist country. The results indicate that basic psychological needs and intrinsic life goals are positively related with subjective well-being but also that extrinsic life goals are positively and highly related with subjective well-being. Furthermore, the orientation toward collectivism is positively related with subjective well-being, suggesting that it is beneficial to be collectivist in a collectivistic country. Finally, the limitations of using predominantly individualistic, Western-developed instruments in Macedonia are discussed.

Moving on, an exploration of character strengths in African Traditional Religion (ATR) is offered by Sahaya G. Selvam and Joanna Collicutt. As the authors write, positive psychology has relied on the world(wide) philosophical and religious traditions for its understanding and classification of core virtues and character strengths and in demonstrating their ubiquity across cultures. However, in this endeavour, reference to African Traditional Religion (ATR) is minimal, and through a qualitative study the authors aim to discern if the ubiquity of character strengths extends to ATR. Among the findings, citizenship and spirituality emerged as stronger themes in ATR, and elderhood rites featured as the most significant anthropological domain. A case is made for the African elder being a cultural paragon of character strengths.

A theoretical exploration of the conception of nature and its impact on well-being is provided by Nicola Rainisio and Paolo Inghilleri, who highlight the great variability of the concept of *nature* across cultures and argue that it could indeed be considered an artefact that contains and conveys cultural information. The cross-cultural research on nature suggests that culture is a valuable theoretical framework to understand the wide range of place-oriented attitudes, emotions and perceptions. Although this is a classic theme in the environmental psychology field, the positive psychological effects triggered by natural environments have been poorly investigated in a cross-cultural perspective, favouring an evolutionary orientation in attempting to settle universal processes. The authors suggest a cross-breeding with some key concepts coming from positive and cultural psychology (optimal experience, flourishing, positive emotions, vitality, cultural self) and propose a wider framework encompassing natural areas, positive place experiences and cultures of belonging.

Finally, Antonella Delle Fave, Ingrid Brdar, Dianne Vella-Brodrick and Marié Wissing provide some findings about the perceived happiness and meaningfulness in the spirituality/religiousness life domain among adults coming from seven Western countries. Participants concurrently evaluated spirituality and religiosity with regards to their perceived levels of happiness and meaningfulness. Results showed significant cross-country differences in happiness and meaningfulness ratings in the spiritual/religious domain. For instance, findings indicated that religion is perceived to be strongly associated with spirituality, but spirituality need not be associated with religion, and that individuals who were high in *spiritual* meaning and happiness were more satisfied with their lives and reported higher *general* meaning and happiness ratings than other participants. The findings further highlight the importance of distinguishing between hedonic and eudaemonic components of well-being, and more specifically between happiness and meaningfulness.

The remaining five chapters of this book prominently investigate well-being across cultures in the light of socio-economic factors. The opening chapter investigates the relationship between South African consumers' living standards and their life satisfaction. Leona Ungerer begins by recognizing how people are bombarded daily with powerful messages that the good life is "the goods life" and how advertisements often imply that happiness and well-being come from attaining wealth and from the purchase and acquisition of goods and services. Indeed, materialism seems to have been singled out as the dominant ideology in modern consumer behaviour, among others leading to the use of possessions as an important measure of personal success. Her findings, collected among participants differing in ethnicity and socio-economic status, showed that purchase decision-makers who had higher objective living standards reported higher satisfaction with life, while across all ethnic groups participants were less satisfied with their lives the lower their incomes were. Differences in life satisfaction were specifically found among consumers from certain ethnic groups. The findings suggest the issue of "what makes a good life" is fraught with cultural assumptions.

Next, Iva Šolcová and Vladimir Kebza discuss the relations between well-being and personality characteristics, values, social desirability, self-concept and self-determining needs in a sample of Czech college students. Their findings highlight a strong association between life satisfaction and self-acceptance and between satisfaction and environmental mastery. Interesting relations were also found between life satisfaction and personality dimensions, basic psychological needs, values, self-construal and social desirability.

In their chapter, Yasumasa Otsuka, Masashi Hori and Junko Kawahito investigate the relationships between income and positive affect, life satisfaction and subjective happiness among Japanese workers. Participants answered a self-reported questionnaire including annual income, positive affect, life satisfaction, subjective happiness and other covariates. The effects of annual income on positive affect, life satisfaction and subjective happiness were subsequently tested, showing no associations between these variables. Potential biases are finally discussed.

The contribution by Pilar Sanjuán and Kristine Jensen de Lopez focuses on the relationships between self-serving attributional bias (SSAB) and subjective well-being in two undergraduate women samples from Denmark and Spain. SSAB has been inversely associated with psychological distress. However, well-being is not merely absence of psychological distress, wherefore positive affect balance and life satisfaction, as components of subjective well-being (SWB), were considered with the aim to explore how SSAB and SWB are related. The results showed that both Danish and Spanish women displayed SSAB. While this bias was greater for the Spanish group, Danish women reported a more positive affect balance and greater life satisfaction. SSAB and the two components of SWB were interrelated in both samples, and mediational analysis showed that positive affect balance mediated the relationships between SSAB and life satisfaction. It is suggested that differences in well-being between the analyzed samples can be explained, at least in part, by socio-economic differences.

Finally, Loredana Ruxandra Gherasim, Simona Butnaru, Alin Gavreliuc and Luminita Mihaela Iacob examine from a cross-cultural perspective the impact of optimistic attributional style and perception of parental behaviour on two educational outcomes: school performance and depression. The effects of ethnic or/and regional differences on these relationships are investigated among Hungarian and Romanian adolescents, as well as among Romanian adolescents living in Moldova. The results indicate both similarities and differences between the ethnic and regional groups. Parental control was a significant predictor of the adolescents' depression and performance, but it did not moderate the relationship between the optimistic attributional style and the adolescents' outcomes. The effects of optimistic attributional style and parental acceptance were moderated by the ethnic/regional group.

The results indicate that the predictors of depression and achievement varied more depending on the regional criterion than the ethnic one. Ethnic differences emerged only when combined with regional differences. Educational implications of the results are also discussed.

As editors of this volume, we feel deeply privileged and grateful to present this collection of scholarly contributions to the public. Positive psychology, now officially well into its second decade, is providing still finer-grained perspectives on the diversity of cultures along with insights about our shared human nature, uniting us for better or worse. Yet, far more important than feeling certain about what is universal and what is cultural specific in the world seems to be our acknowledgement of cultural diversity – at least in the many forms respecting basic human needs for stable, loving relationships; for personal flourishing through play, learning and creativity; and for personal freedom under social responsibility – as essentially enriching in itself and thereby making global unity truly meaningful. The quality of our future seems to depend on good *combinations* of cultural diversity and human unity, indeed maybe more so than anything else. Moreover, with a bit of good will, most of us could probably agree on such an ideal as indeed inherently spiritual, as a certain belief in life before death.

References

Acerbi, A., Enquist, M., & Ghirlanda, S. (2009). Cultural evolution and individual development of openness and conservatism. *PNAS, 106*, 18931–18935.

Bateson, P. P., & Hinde, R. A. (Eds.). (1976). *Growing points in ethology*. London: Cambridge University Press.

Bakker, A., Killmer, C., Siegrist, J., & Schaufeli, W. (2000). Effort-reward imbalance and burnout among nurses. *Journal of Advanced Nursing, 31*, 884–891.

Becker, D., & Marecek, J. (2008). Positive psychology: History in the remaking? *Theory & Psychology, 18*, 591–604.

Berger, P. L., & Luckman, T. (1966). *The social construction of reality*. New York: Doubleday & Co.

Boyd, R., Richerson, P. J., & Henrich, J. (2011). The cultural niche: Why social learning is essential for human adaptation. *PNAS, 108*(Suppl 2), 10918–10925.

Christopher, J. C., & Hickinbottom, S. (2008). Positive psychology, ethnocentrism, and the disguised ideology of individualism. *Theory & Psychology, 18*, 563–589.

Delle Fave, A., & Bassi, M. (2009). Sharing optimal experiences and promoting good community life in a multicultural society. *The Journal of Positive Psychology, 4*, 280–289.

Delle Fave, A., Brdar, I., Freire, T., Vella-Brodrick, D., & Wissing, M. (2011a). The eudaimonic and hedonic components of happiness: Qualitative and quantitative findings. *Social Indicators Research, 100*, 158–207.

Delle Fave, A., Massimini, F., & Bassi, M. (2011b). *Psychological selection and optimal experience across cultures: Social empowerment through personal growth*. Dordrecht: Springer.

Diamond, J. (1997). *Guns, germs, and steel. The fates of human societies*. New York: W.W. Norton & Co.

Diener, E. (Ed.). (2009). *Culture and well-being*. Dordrecht: Springer.

Diener, E., Oishi, S., & Lucas, R. (2003). Personality, culture, and subjective well-being: Emotional and cognitive evaluations of life. *Annual Review of Psychology, 54*, 403–425.

Fischer, R. (2009). Where is culture in cross-cultural research? *International Journal of Cross-Cultural Management, 9*, 25–49.

Fischer, R., Vauclair, C. M., Fontaine, J. R. I., & Schwartz, S. H. (2010). Are individual-level and country-level value structures different? Testing Hofstede's legacy with the Schwartz value survey. *Journal of Cross-Cultural Psychology, 41*, 135–151.

Freeman, M., & Brockmeier, J. (2001). Narrative integrity: Autobiographical identity and the meaning of the "good life". In J. Brockmeier & D. Carbaugh (Eds.), *Narrative and identity: Studies in autobiography, self, and culture* (pp. 75–99). Amsterdam: John Benjamins Publishing Co.

Gavin, J., & Mason, R. (2004). The virtuous organization: The value of happiness in the workplace. *Organizational Dynamics, 33*, 379–392.

Henrich, J., Boyd, R., & Richerson, P. J. (2008). Five misunderstandings about cultural evolution. *Human Nature, 19*, 119–137.

Hofstede, G., Bond, M. H., & Luk, C. L. (1993). Individual perceptions of organizational cultures: A methodological treatise on levels of analysis. *Organization Studies, 14*, 483–503.

Inglehart, R., & Baker, W. E. (2000). Modernization, cultural change and the persistence of traditional values. *American Sociological Review, 65*, 19–51.

Jablonka, E., & Lamb, M. J. (2005). *Evolution in four dimensions. Genetic, epigenetic, behavioural and symbolic variations in the history of life*. Cambridge, MA: MIT Press.

Kirkman, B. L., Lowe, K. B., & Gibson, C. (2006). A quarter century of culture's consequences: A review of empirical research incorporating Hofstede's cultural values framework. *Journal of International Business Studies, 37*, 285–320.

Kristjansson, K. (2010). Positive psychology, happiness, and virtue: The troublesome conceptual issues. *Review of General Psychology, 14*, 296–310.

Laland, K. N., Odling-Smee, J., & Feldman, M. W. (2000). Niche construction, biological evolution, and cultural change. *The Behavioral and Brain Sciences, 23*, 131–146.

Leung, K., & Bond, M. H. (2004). Social axioms: A model for social beliefs in multicultural perspective. *Advances in Experimental Social Psychology, 36*, 119–197.

Lu, L., & Gilmour, R. (2006). Individual-oriented and socially oriented cultural conceptions of subjective well-being: Conceptual analysis and scale development. *Asian Journal of Social Psychology, 9*, 36–49.

Maslach, C., & Goldberg, J. (1998). Prevention of burnout: New perspectives. *Applied and Preventive Psychology, 7*, 63–74.

Maslach, C., Schaufeli, W., & Leiter, M. (2001). Job burnout. *Annual Review of Psychology, 52*, 397–422.

Massimini, F., & Delle Fave, A. (2000). Individual development in a bio-cultural perspective. *American Psychologist, 55*, 24–33.

Na, J., Grossmann, I., Varnum, E. W., Kitayama, S., Gonzalez, R., & Nisbett, R. E. (2010). Cultural differences are not always reducible to individual differences. *PNAS, 107*, 6192–6197.

Newson, L., Richerson, P. J., & Boyd, R. (2007). Cultural evolution and the shaping of cultural diversity. In S. Kitayama & D. Cohen (Eds.), *Handbook of cultural psychology* (pp. 454–476). New York: Guilford Press.

Oishi, S., Kesebir, S., & Snyder, B. H. (2009). Sociology: A lost connection in social psychology. *Personality and Social Psychology Review, 13*, 334–353.

Park, N., Peterson, C., & Seligman, M. E. P. (2006). Character strengths in fifty-four nations and the fifty US states. *The Journal of Positive Psychology, 1*, 118–129.

Peterson, C., & Seligman, M. E. P. (2004). *Character strengths and virtues. A handbook and classification*. New York: Oxford University Press.

Richardson, F. C., & Guignon, C. B. (2008). Positive psychology and philosophy of social science. *Theory & Psychology, 18*, 605–627.

Richerson, P. J., & Boyd, R. (2005). *Not by genes alone. How culture transformed human evolution*. Chicago: University of Chicago Press.

Sauter, D. A., Eisner, F., Ekman, P., & Scott, S. K. (2010). Cross-cultural recognition of basic emotions through non-verbal emotional vocalizations. *PNAS, 107*, 2408–2412.

Schwartz, S. H. (1992). Universals in the content and structure of values: Theoretical advances and empirical tests in 20 countries. *Advances in Experimental Social Psychology, 25*, 1–65.

Schwartz, S. H. (2006). A theory of cultural value orientations: Explication and applications. *Comparative Sociology, 5*, 136–182.

Slife, B. D., & Richardson, F. C. (2008). Problematic ontological underpinnings of positive psychology. *Theory & Psychology, 18*, 699–723.

Super, C. M., & Harkness, S. (1986). The developmental niche: A conceptualization at the interface of child and culture. *International Journal of Behavioral Development, 9*, 545–569.

Strimling, P., Enquist, M., & Eriksson, K. (2009). Repeated learning makes cultural evolution unique. *PNAS, 108*, 13870–13874.

Tafarodi, R. W., Bonn, G., Liang, H., Takai J., Moriizumi S., Belhekar, V., & Padhye, A. (2011). What makes for a good life? A four-nation study. *Journal of Happiness Studies*, Online First, 19 August 2011. DOI 10.1007/s10902-011-9290-6.

Vaalsiner, J. (1998). *The guided mind*. Cambridge, MA: Harvard University Press.

Vaalsiner, J. (2007). Personal culture and conduct of value. *Journal of Social, Evolutionary, and Cultural Psychology, 1*, 59–65.

Veenhoven, R. (2010). *World database of happiness, collection happiness in nations*. Rotterdam: Erasmus University. http://www1.eur.nl/fsw/happiness/ Accessed January 4, 2012

Chapter 2
VIA Character Strengths: Research and Practice (The First 10 Years)

Ryan M. Niemiec

Introduction

The VIA Classification and VIA Inventory of Strengths are widely used by researchers and practitioners around the world. This work with character strengths is one of the most substantial initiatives to emerge from the burgeoning science of positive psychology to date. Research on the VIA Classification (Peterson and Seligman 2004) is flourishing, and practitioners ranging from psychologists and coaches to business leaders and educators are eager to find ways to apply the research to their practices while maintaining prudence with the findings. That said, applied research on the 24 character strengths – their use in practice, the effect of strength combinations, and the outcomes of each – is fairly new territory.

There has been a strong interest in applying the research on character strengths across disciplines, as evidenced in positive psychotherapy (Seligman et al. 2006); various forms of coaching, ranging from executive to life, health, and parent coaching; use with children, adolescents, teachers, and school systems (Fox Eades 2008; Park and Peterson 2009b); in positive education (Geelong Grammer School in Australia); positive institutions, business, and Appreciative Inquiry (Cooperrider 2009; Cooperrider and Whitney 2005); and faculty development and teaching (McGovern and Miller 2008).

The VIA Classification

The creation of the VIA Classification of Character Strengths and Virtues was funded by the Manuel D. and Rhoda Mayerson Foundation in 2000. This work emerged from several scientific meetings led by Martin E. P. Seligman and rigorous

R.M. Niemiec, Psy.D. (✉)
VIA Institute on Character, 312 Walnut St., Suite 3600, Cincinnati, OH, 45202, USA
e-mail: ryan@viacharacter.org

H.H. Knoop and A. Delle Fave (eds.), *Well-Being and Cultures: Perspectives from Positive Psychology*, Cross-Cultural Advancements in Positive Psychology 3, DOI 10.1007/978-94-007-4611-4_2, © Springer Science+Business Media Dordrecht 2013

Table 2.1 The VIA classification of character strengths and Virtues

Wisdom	*Creativity*: originality, adaptivity, ingenuity
	Curiosity: interest, novelty-seeking, exploration, openness to experience
	Judgment: Critical thinking, thinking things through, open-mindedness
	Love of learning: mastering new skills and topics, systematically adding to knowledge
	Perspective: wisdom, providing wise counsel, taking the big picture view
Courage	*Bravery*: valor, not shrinking from fear, speaking up for what's right
	Perseverance: persistence, industry, finishing what one starts
	Honesty: authenticity, integrity
	Zest: vitality, enthusiasm, vigor, energy, feeling alive and activated
Humanity	*Love*: both loving and being loved, valuing close relations with others
	Kindness: generosity, nurturance, care, compassion, altruism, "niceness"
	Social/emotional intelligence: being aware of the motives/feelings of self/others, knowing what makes other people tick
Justice	*Teamwork*: citizenship, social responsibility, loyalty
	Fairness: just, not letting feelings bias decisions about others
	Leadership: organizing group activities, encouraging a group to get things done
Temperance	*Forgiveness*: mercy, accepting others' shortcomings, giving people a second chance
	Humility: modesty, letting one's accomplishments speak for themselves
	Prudence: careful, cautious, not taking undue risks
	Self-regulation: self-control, discipline, managing impulses and emotions
Transcendence	*Appreciation of beauty and excellence*: awe, wonder, elevation
	Gratitude: thankful for the good, expressing thanks, feeling blessed
	Hope: optimism, future-mindedness, future orientation
	Humor: playfulness, bringing smiles to others, lightheartedness
	Spirituality: religiousness, faith, purpose, meaning

historical analysis led by Christopher Peterson, who collaborated with 53 other leading scientists over a period of 3 years. The result was a comprehensive typology. Six virtues – wisdom, courage, humanity, justice, temperance, and transcendence – were identified as core characteristics valued by moral philosophers and religious thinkers across time and world cultures (Peterson and Seligman 2004). Twenty-four corresponding strengths of character – "psychological ingredients" or pathways to those virtues – emerged out of a lengthy list of candidates that were thoroughly examined. The complete list of virtues and strengths is reported in Table 2.1. In addition to being measurable and ubiquitous across cultures, each strength needed to meet most of the following ten criteria: fulfilling, morally valued, does not diminish others, has non-felicitous opposites, trait-like, distinctive from other strengths, has paragons who exemplify it, has prodigies, selective absence of it in some situations, and has institutions/rituals to celebrate or express it (Peterson and Seligman 2004).

Character strengths and virtues have been determined to be universal across cultures, nations, and belief systems (Dahlsgaard et al. 2005; Park et al. 2006) and readily found in some of the most remote areas on the planet (Biswas-Diener 2006).

They are remarkably similar across 54 nations and across the United States (Park et al. 2006).

Character strengths are substantially stable, universal personality traits that manifest through thinking (cognition), feeling (affect), willing (conation or volition), and action (behavior). They are morally valued and are beneficial to oneself and others. These positive psychological characteristics are considered to be the basic building blocks of human goodness and human flourishing (Peterson and Seligman 2004). As originally hypothesized by Seligman and Csikszentmihalyi (2000), positive character traits occupy a central role in the field of positive psychology. Pleasure, flow, and other positive experiences are enabled by good character (Park and Peterson 2009a; Peterson et al. 2007). The VIA Classification is descriptive, not prescriptive; it was created to thoroughly examine and describe what is best in human beings. It is not based on any particular theory, thus cannot be called a taxonomy of strengths.

Character strengths are moderately heritable, and twin studies show that love, humor, modesty, and teamwork are most influenced by environmental factors (Steger et al. 2007).

Prevalence

The most commonly endorsed character strengths reported are (in descending order) kindness, fairness, honesty, gratitude, and judgment, while the least endorsed character strengths are prudence, modesty, and self-regulation (Park et al. 2006). Similarly, the most prevalent character strengths in a UK sample were judgment, fairness, curiosity, love of learning, and kindness (Linley et al. 2007).

Young adults (ages 18–24) from the USA and Japan showed similar distributions of VIA strengths – higher strengths of kindness, humor, and love and lower strengths of prudence, modesty, and self-regulation; in addition, females reported more kindness and love, while males reported more bravery and creativity (Shimai et al. 2006). When compared with US adults, youth from the USA are higher on the character strengths of hope, teamwork, and zest, and adults are higher on appreciation of beauty and excellence, honesty, leadership, and open-mindedness (Park and Peterson 2006b). The most prevalent character strengths in very young children are love, kindness, creativity, curiosity, and humor (Park and Peterson 2006a).

Among two military samples (US and Norway), the highest strengths were honesty, hope, bravery, perseverance, and teamwork, and the two samples correlated higher with one another than with a civilian sample (Matthews et al. 2006).

The VIA Survey

The VIA Inventory of Strengths (often referred to as the VIA Survey, or VIA-IS; see www.viasurvey.org) – a measurement instrument designed to assess the 24 character strengths – has been taken by well over a million people and is a free, online tool. The VIA-IS has good reliability and validity. The results agree with reports by friends and family members of those who complete the test. The tool has been used extensively by researchers studying the correlates and outcomes of various character strengths; much of this research has been published in peer-reviewed scientific journals, satisfying the gold standard of scientific research. For the assessment of character strengths in children/adolescents between the ages of 10 and 17, there is the widely used, validated VIA Youth Survey (Park and Peterson 2006b). Additional briefer youth surveys have been developed and are currently being studied.

The VIA-IS has been translated in Danish, French, German, Spanish, and simplified Chinese and is in a later stage of the translation process in more than 20 other languages, including Urdu, Farsi, and Portuguese.

At times, the question is raised as to the impact of VIA Survey-takers attempting to "look good" in their responses to the items. The Marlowe-Crowne Social Desirability Index is used to evaluate the potential impact of this phenomenon; the only character strength scale scores that correlate significantly with social desirability are prudence and spirituality. Such biases are reduced by anonymous administration and the use of computerized tests, both of which are typically part of the VIA-IS.

Several studies have conducted factor analyses, and further analyses are currently being conducted. In general, these results show strong consistency with the VIA Classification. One factor analysis found the 24 character strengths were well represented by both a one- and four-factor solution in which significant relationships were found between each of the 24 character strengths, the one- and four-factor solutions, and the Five Factor Model of personality. The four factors were described as positivity, intellect, conscientiousness, and niceness (Macdonald et al. 2008). Another factor analysis found five factors: interpersonal (humor, kindness, leadership, love, social intelligence, and teamwork), fortitude (bravery, honesty, judgment, perseverance, perspective, and self-regulation), cognitive (appreciation of beauty/excellence, creativity, curiosity, and love of learning), transcendence (gratitude, hope, religiousness, and zest), and temperance (fairness, forgiveness, modesty/humility, and prudence) (Peterson et al. 2008). A third factor analysis found four factors: interpersonal, which reflects positive behavior toward others; fortitude, which reflects openness and bravery; vitality, which reflects a global factor of positive qualities; and cautiousness, which reflects self-control (Brdar and Kashdan 2010). In general, it appears that the interpersonal strengths within the justice and humanity virtues converge, that zest might better locate under transcendence, and that humor loads more strongly under wisdom or humanity. Several other factor analyses have found comparable results, including Littman-Ovadia and Lavy (in press), Shryack et al. (2010), Singh and Choubisa (2010), and Ruch et al. (2010). Studies using much larger sample sizes and different statistical procedures are currently underway (see www.viacharacter.org).

Conceptualization of "Character"

The work on the VIA expands the thinking on what is meant by the word character, which has different meanings within and among cultures. Traditional views of character typically identify a few character traits and espouse that every person should strive to develop this core set of characteristics as much as possible. Other approaches to character consider it to be either present or absent and not occurring in degrees.

The creation of a universal language for what is best in people opens the door to a variety of important principles that lay the groundwork for the science of character:

- Character is individualized and idiosyncratic. Each individual has a unique profile of character strengths.
- Character is plural (Peterson and Seligman 2004). Individuals are not simply honest or kind, brave or wise, and humble or fair; rather, an individual's character is best understood as a profile of strengths.
- Character strengths have structure, depth, and dimensionality. People are high or low on different strengths of character, and certain profiles are more typical than others.
- Character strengths are elemental. Character strengths are the basic building blocks of goodness in the individual. They are the core parts of the personality that account for us being our best selves. These elements can combine to form complex character strengths.
- Character strengths are shaped by context and expressed in situations (Schwartz and Sharpe 2006). In the social context, one individual might call forth her social intelligence and curiosity; when eating, use self-regulation and prudence; at work, persistence and teamwork; and with family, use love and kindness.
- Character strengths are expressed in degrees. Individuals will likely express their character strengths in different ways and to a greater or lesser extent based on the circumstance they are in. The level or amount of kindness expressed to the person's relationship partner (e.g., offering to cook dinner) differs in scope from that expressed to a homeless person on the street (e.g., giving away $5); also, the individual might find it very easy to express kindness to fellow employees and very difficult in another work situation, such as while communicating with a supervisor.
- Character strengths are interactive and interdependent. It is likely that in most situations individuals will express a combination of character strengths together (curiosity and creativity) rather than one character strength alone. Therefore, there are dynamics that occur as the strengths interact with one another, as they lead to increases in one another or as they hinder the expression of one another. Also, character strengths are interdependent – it is difficult to express kindness without some level of humility or to be perseverant without some degree of self-regulation.

- Character strengths are substantially stable but can and do change. Character strengths are part of an individual's personality and may change in response to important life events or as a result of deliberate interventions or conscious lifestyle actions.
- Balanced expression of character strengths is critical. Character strengths can easily be overused and underused. Optimal strengths use occurs according to the golden mean of character strengths, originally derived from Aristotle (2000) – the right combination of strengths, expressed to the right degree, and in the right situation.

Character Strengths: Empirical Research

Character Strengths and Life Satisfaction

Probably the most common variable studied in positive psychology is life satisfaction (happiness). This is true for research on character strengths, which has found a strong connection between character strengths and life satisfaction. Here are some specifics:

Five character strengths show a consistent, robust relationship to life satisfaction: hope, zest, gratitude, curiosity, and love (Park et al. 2004). This has been replicated a number of times; for example, similar results can be found among Swiss, Germans, Austrians (Ruch et al. 2007), Croatians (Brdar and Kashdan 2010), and young Japanese adults (Shimai et al. 2006).

The character strengths least related to life satisfaction (weak association) are modesty/humility, creativity, appreciation of beauty and excellence, judgment, and love of learning (Park et al. 2004). Viewed from another angle, it has been found that the strengths of the "heart" (e.g., love, gratitude) are more strongly associated with well-being than are strengths of the "head" (e.g., creativity, judgment, appreciation of beauty and excellence; Park and Peterson 2008b; Park et al. 2004).

Seligman's (2002) theory of authentic happiness addresses three pathways to happiness: pleasure, engagement, and meaning. A life orientation that encompasses all three pathways is associated with life satisfaction and might be viewed as "the full life" (Peterson et al. 2007). While each pathway has been found to be a distinct pathway and to predict happiness, the pursuit of meaning and engagement is more predictive of life satisfaction than the pursuit of pleasure (Peterson et al. 2006; Vella-Brodrick et al. 2009). In a study of nations, three groups emerged in a study of 27 nations and routes to happiness: nations high in pleasure and engagement; those high in engagement and meaning; and those low in pleasure, engagement, and meaning. Nations highest in each route were South Africa (pleasure), Switzerland (engagement), and South Korea (meaning; Park et al. 2009). These findings are interesting to consider in light of those character strengths that correlate highest with each authentic-happiness pathway. The character strengths most associated with the *meaning* route to happiness are religiousness, gratitude, hope, zest, and curiosity; those most associated with the *engagement* route to happiness are zest, curiosity, hope, perseverance, and perspective; and those most associated with the *pleasure* route to happiness are humor, zest, hope, social intelligence, and love (Peterson et al. 2007).

Among youth, the character strengths most related to life satisfaction are love, gratitude, hope, and zest; very young children (ages 3–9) described by their parents as happy are also noted as showing love, hope, and zest (Park and Peterson 2009b). A parent's strength of self-regulation is strongly associated with his or her child's life satisfaction but not the parent's own (Park and Peterson 2006a).

A higher total score of all 24 character strengths on the VIA-IS correlates positively with life satisfaction and indicates that strong character is associated with happiness and the good life (Ruch et al. 2007).

Character strength predictors of satisfaction in college were hope, social intelligence, self-regulation, and fairness (Lounsbury et al. 2009).

Character Strengths and Health and Wellness

When an individual has a physical disorder, there is less of a toll on life satisfaction if the person ranks high on the character strengths of bravery, kindness, and humor. For psychological disorders, there is less of a toll on life satisfaction if they rank high on the character strengths of appreciation of beauty and excellence and love of learning (Park et al. 2006).

A handful of studies have found a health benefit to the strength of gratitude. The practice of counting blessings was linked to fewer physical symptoms, more optimistic life appraisals, more time exercising, improved well-being, and optimal functioning (Emmons and McCullough 2003). Adolescent students who counted blessings reported higher levels of optimism and life satisfaction, less negative affect, and fewer physical symptoms (Froh et al. 2008). The practice of gratitude was linked to increases in well-being among those with neuromuscular disease (Emmons and McCullough 2003).

In terms of sexual health, some character strengths were associated with lower levels of sexual behaviors and sex-related beliefs among African–American adolescents. Specifically on the VIA, higher love of learning was related to boys' self-reported abstinence from sexual intercourse and boys' and girls' self-reported abstinence from drug use, higher curiosity was related to boys' and girls' belief in no premarital sex (love of learning was also significant for boys), prudence was related to reported abstinence from sexual intimacy, and judgment was related to sexual initiation efficacy for girls and boys (leadership was also significant for girls; Ma et al. 2008).

There have been few studies looking at the role of character strengths and adherence issues. One exception found hope to be a significant predictor of medication adherence among asthma patients between ages 8 and 12 (Berg et al. 2007).

Character Strengths and Achievement

In terms of achievement in work and school, perseverance appears to be the most robust character strength, emerging in most studies conducted in areas related to life success. Perseverance, love, gratitude, and hope predicted academic achievement in middle school students and college students (Park and Peterson 2009a). After controlling for IQ, strengths of perseverance, fairness, gratitude, honesty, hope, and perspective predicted GPA (Park and Peterson 2008a). In another study, those character strengths that predicted GPA in college students were perseverance, love of learning, humor, fairness, and kindness (Lounsbury et al. 2009). Higher hope levels are related to greater scholastic and social competence and to creativity levels (Onwuegbuzie 1999).

Effective teachers (judged by the gains of their students on standardized tests) are those who are high in social intelligence, zest, and humor in a longitudinal study (reported in Park and Peterson 2009a). Military performance among West Point cadets was predicted by the character strength of love (Peterson and Park 2009).

Character Strengths and Psychological Problems

The character strength of hope appears to be a key factor in this area. Hope, zest, and leadership were substantially related to fewer problems with anxiety and depression (Park and Peterson 2008a). Hope is negatively related to indicators of psychological distress and school maladjustment (internalizing and externalizing behaviors; Gilman et al. 2006). Persistence, honesty, prudence, and love were substantially related to fewer externalizing problems such as aggression (Park and Peterson 2008a).

In terms of trauma, the more traumatic events an individual reports, the higher the character strength scores (with the exception of gratitude, hope, and love; Peterson et al. 2008). Hope, kindness, social intelligence, self-regulation, and perspective buffer against the negative effects of stress and trauma (Park and Peterson 2006c, 2009a). Gratitude, hope, kindness, leadership, love, spirituality, and teamwork all increased in a US sample (but not a European sample) 2 months after the September 11, 2001, attack on the World Trade Center in New York City; 10 months after September 11, these character strengths were still elevated but to a lesser degree (Peterson and Seligman 2003). The various dimensions of posttraumatic growth appear to correspond with particular character strengths: improved relationships with others (kindness, love), openness to new possibilities (curiosity, creativity, love of learning), greater appreciation of life (appreciation of beauty, gratitude, zest), enhanced personal strength (bravery, honesty, perseverance), and spiritual development (religiousness; Peterson et al. 2008; Tedeschi and Calhoun 1995).

Character Strengths: Additional Research

Reviewing all of the correlations, consequences, enabling factors, inhibiting factors, and related research on each of the 24 character strengths over the decades is not feasible for this article.

Here are some of the recent highlights:

- Viewing one's work as a "calling," in which one's work is viewed as a source of fulfillment that is socially useful and personal meaningful, rather than as merely a job that pays the bills or solely as a pathway for career advancement, is predicted by the character strength of zest (Peterson et al. 2009).
- Grateful individuals report higher positive mood, optimism, life satisfaction, vitality, religiousness and spirituality, and less depression and envy than less grateful individuals. Grateful people also tend to be more helpful, supportive, forgiving, empathic, and agreeable (McCullough et al. 2002).
- In a study of nearly 1,200 kids who wore a beeping watch prompting them to write about their thoughts, feelings, and actions eight times per day, the most curious kids were compared with the bored kids (the top 207 and the bottom 207). The curious were more optimistic, hopeful, confident, and had a higher sense of self-determination and self-efficacy, believing they were in control of their actions and decisions, than the bored kids who felt like pawns with no control of their destiny (Hunter and Csikszentmihalyi 2003).
- Military leaders' character strength of humor predicted their followers' trust, while followers' character strength of perspective earned their leaders' trust (Sweeney et al. 2009).
- Popular students, as identified by teacher ratings, are more likely to score highly on civic strengths such as leadership and fairness, and temperance strengths of self-regulation, prudence, and forgiveness. Interestingly, none of the humanity strengths, such as love and kindness, were related to popularity (Park and Peterson 2009b).

Character Strengths: Practical Applications

General Approach

Many practitioners find that working with a client's character strengths is one of the most exciting and fulfilling areas of their work. At the same time, there is no unifying theory or consensus on how a practitioner must proceed in this work. Following this general approach, I will focus on some of the more recent findings that inform practitioners interested in applying the latest science in their work with clients. I hope practitioners will approach these findings with a sense of prudence by viewing them as forward movements with long terrain ahead, rather than as absolute truths or the final answer. What follows is only a sampling of some of the findings and theoretical contributions over the last decade.

To simplify the various strength-based approaches and summarize the approach practitioners take when working with character strengths, Niemiec (2009) offered the three-step process of aware, explore, and apply. The practitioner helps the client become *more* aware of their existing character strengths, which is a critical task as

Linley (2008) has reported that fewer than one-third of individuals have a meaningful understanding of their strengths. The practitioner follows this with questions that help the client dig deep in exploring their strengths – addressing when they have previously used strengths at their best and worst and how they might tap into strengths to create a best possible future. Exploration is followed by the application of an action plan or goal targeted to improve a particular strength. Looking to character strength exemplars in one's life and in the movies (Niemiec and Wedding 2008) is ideal for rallying this stage through the power of observational learning (Bandura 1986). In addition to the aware-explore-apply model, a number of additional strength-based models can be applied to character strengths practice including models from coaching (e.g., the GROW model), business (the Appreciative Inquiry model), and social-constructivist psychology (the 4 Es model; Wong 2006).

As the steps are implemented and repeated, it is optimal that strength spotting (Linley 2008) be used throughout the three phases of the model. A preliminary step involving resource priming (Fluckiger and Gross Holtforth 2008) should also be considered; this involves the practitioner focusing on the client's strengths prior to the session. When working with helping clients explore and apply character strengths – strengths development interventions – there are a number of issues to be attuned to, such as considering how strengths work together toward a desired outcome, novel ways to use strengths, the strength-environment fit, the liabilities of strengths, the modulation of strengths to situational demands by using them more or less, and how they align with values (Louis 2011). In addition, the golden mean of strengths – finding the right balance of strength expression in the right context so as not to be overplayed or underplayed – is of great importance for practitioners (Biswas-Diener et al. 2011; Linley 2008).

The VIA PRO Report (and its accompanying Practitioner's Guide) is an interpretive report that provides a close look at the individual's character strengths through the use of five graphs, description of key research around certain character strengths, ways to explore strengths, a description of the overuse and underuse of their highest strengths, and a description of the most recent interventions for building or expressing each of the 24 character strengths (see www.viapros.org/www/). Practitioners have found this to be particularly helpful as a "best practice" tool for working with strengths and it serves as a jump-start in the early stages of practitioner-client relationships.

Signature Strengths

The quintessential exercise in working with character strength has become the suggestion to use a signature strength in a new and unique way. Signature strengths are character strengths that are displayed the majority of time in relevant settings, readily named and owned by the individual, and are easily recognized by others as characteristic of the individual (Peterson and Seligman 2004). Seligman (2002) added that signature strengths have a rapid learning curve, are invigorating to use, involve a sense of authenticity ("this is the real me") when used, and involve intrinsic motivation. While the convention has been that people typically name between 3 and 7 strengths of the 24 VIA strengths as signature, this is only a general rule of thumb, and research is currently ongoing to determine how many signature strengths individuals typically have. Finding new and unique ways to use signature strengths is indeed an effective intervention; it increased happiness and decreased depression for 6 months in a large, randomized, controlled trial on the Internet (Seligman et al. 2005). In the same sample, a suggestion to write down three positive things that happened during the day (increasing the strength of gratitude) led to similar results over the 6-month period. These results have been replicated at least one time with similar significant effects on increasing happiness for 6 months and lowering depression for either 3 or 6 months (Mongrain and Anselmo 2009).

Another randomly controlled study assigned individuals to a group instructed to use two signature strengths, to a group instructed to use one signature strength and one bottom strength, or to a control group. Results revealed significant gains in satisfaction with life for both treatment groups compared to controls, but there were no differences between the two treatment groups (Rust et al. 2009). Both treatment groups wrote about an event or occurrence in the past when they successfully used their character strength. Each week, they also wrote about a plan or situation for the coming week in which they could apply the strength. Another signature-strength study found that the use of one's top strengths led to a decreased likelihood of depression and stress and an increase in satisfaction in law students (Peterson and Peterson 2008). Finding novel ways to use signature strengths was a core part of a coaching program for youth that led to increases in the students' self-reported levels of engagement and hope (Madden et al. 2011). In another study, Mitchell et al. (2009) asked participants to develop three of their top ten strengths and find ways to develop them in their daily life and found benefits to the cognitive component of well-being at 3 months.

Deployment of character strengths in the work setting was linked with greater well-being, vocational satisfaction, and meaning (Littman-Ovadia and Davidovitch 2010; Littman-Ovadia and Steger 2010). While it is important to endorse one's strengths, these studies show it is important to take it to the next step and deploy them at work. In the first study to explore the connections between signature strengths use, goal progress, psychological needs, and well-being, Linley et al. (2010) found that those who used their signature strengths made more progress on their goals, met their basic psychological needs (autonomy, relatedness, and competence), and were higher in overall well-being (a combination of higher life satisfaction, higher positive emotions, and lower negative emotions). This study helps pave the way in explaining why working on signature strengths leads to greater well-being.

Wisdom Strengths

These are the cognitive strengths of creativity, curiosity, judgment, love of learning, and perspective. Most creativity training programs work, especially when divergent thinking – the capacity to generate multiple alternative solutions as opposed to one correct solution – is fostered (Scott et al. 2004). Many interventions help to increase creativity in older adults, such as cultural/art programs (e.g., music, dance, drawing), poetry, journaling, problem-solving activities, reminiscence, and psychoeducational groups (Flood and Phillips 2007).

In an experiment in which participants were instructed to pay attention to three novel features with something they disliked (i.e., use their curiosity), the participants changed the way they viewed the activity, and weeks later they were more likely to have done the task again on their own (Langer 2005). Individuals are more likely to engage in active open-mindedness of multiple views (i.e., judgment) when asked to make decisions around values/goals that are both strong and conflicting (Tetlock 1986). Students are more likely to value and enjoy learning if they're achieving their grade goal, the subject matter is of personal interest, or the reasons for learning are task-oriented (e.g., there are markers for how they can improve; Covington 1999).

There are three major paths for developing wisdom (perspective): learning from mentors and reading philosophical literature, teaching skills and wise patterns of thinking and decision making, and using direct, short-term interventions, such as imagined conversation and imagined travel (Glück and Baltes 2006).

Courage Strengths

These are the emotional strengths of bravery, perseverance, honesty, and zest. Labeling one's actions in retrospect as courageous can lead to or promote courage or at least positive states and values that lead to courageous behaviors (Finfgeld 1999; Hannah et al. 2007). Most people have tried to increase their courage/bravery in some way. Pury (2008) looked at the strategies people employ to increase courage. The most common approach was outcome-focused strategies in which individuals thought of the outcome of the courageous act – thinking of the person being helped, reminding themselves that it was the right thing to do, or remembering that there was an obligation to act. The second most common approach can be categorized as emotion-focused coping, which involves individuals reminding themselves to not fear, receiving encouragement from others, and keeping a positive focus. The least common approach was problem-focused coping, in which individuals reminded themselves of the action or mentally rehearsed their plans for the brave act.

Honesty, empathy, and courage – conceptualized as academic heroism – predicted academic honesty and are noted as three potential routes for developing heroism and virtues (Staats et al. 2008). Reinforcement of high effort on tasks results in transfer of effort to other tasks (greater perseverance; Eisenberger 1992; Hickman et al. 1998).

Potential pathways for increasing zest, particularly in the workplace, may be to cultivate optimism, gratitude, or savoring; emphasize good social relationships outside work; and focus on physical health and fitness (Peterson et al. 2009).

Humanity Strengths

These are the interpersonal strengths of love, kindness, and social intelligence. The focus on cultivating love toward oneself and/or others was found to increase feelings of social connection and positivity toward others (Hutcherson et al. 2008), as well as positive emotions, sense of purpose, and mindfulness in general (Fredrickson et al. 2008). The approach of sharing good news (capitalization) with a person who responds in an active, enthusiastic, genuine, and positive way (active-constructive responding) is beneficial for the speaker, the listener, and their relationship (Gable et al. 2004). Shelly Gable, the lead researcher in this area, has shared that the key character strengths involved in this process are love, social intelligence, and self-regulation (Gable, 2009, personal communication). Kindness and gratitude increased among happy Japanese women who counted their kind acts (Otake et al. 2006).

Justice Strengths

These are the civic strengths of teamwork, fairness, and leadership. Potential pathways to build teamwork and develop successful teams come from correlational research that found that team optimism predicts outcomes for teams that are newly formed; and team resiliency and team efficacy predict outcomes for established teams (West et al. 2009). Instructors are more likely to be perceived as fair if they present information clearly, give regular feedback, stick to the course syllabus, and give many opportunities to earn a good grade in the course (Chory 2007). Moral-reasoning development (fairness) is developed through stimulating and interactive peer discussions that involve moral issues, heterogeneous reasoning, and orientation toward consensus or resolution of disagreement (also called transactive discussions; Berkowtiz and Gibbs 1983). The development of two or three different leadership styles (e.g., directive, participative, coaching) relates to higher leader behavioral flexibility, which is an important characteristic of effective leaders (Sumner-Armstrong et al. 2008).

Temperance Strengths

These are the protective strengths of forgiveness, modesty/humility, prudence, and self-regulation. Writing about the personal benefits of forgiving a transgressor led to greater forgiveness than writing about the traumatic features of a transgression suffered or an unrelated control topic (McCullough et al. 2006). Viewing and working with forgiveness as a process, whether this is done individually or in groups, is crucial for building this strength (Baskin and Enright 2004). A meta-analysis of 65 group-intervention conditions found that the amount of time spent for empathizing with transgressors, committing to forgive, and practical strategies (e.g., anger management and relaxation) was significantly related to forgiveness outcome (Wade et al. 2005).

Daily self-control exercises increase a general core capacity for self-control (i.e., our self-regulation "muscle"), such as food monitoring, improving mood, improving posture, physical exercise programs, financial monitoring exercises, and the use of a non-preferred hand to do routine activities (Baumeister et al. 2006).

Transcendence Strengths

These are the spiritual strengths of appreciation of beauty/excellence, gratitude, hope, humor, and religiousness/spirituality. Keeping a "beauty log" of writing briefly about the beauty one appreciates in nature, art, or morality leads to a higher engagement with moral beauty and trait hope levels (Diessner et al. 2006). A combination of cognitive strategies (e.g., evaluating beliefs) and social problem-solving strategies (e.g., assertiveness training) leads to greater optimism (Gillham et al. 1995). Visualizing and writing about one's best possible self at a time in the future leads to increases in optimism/hope and well-being (King 2001; Sheldon and Lyubomirsky 2006).

Emmons (2007; Emmons and McCullough 2003) reviews a number of strategies for building gratitude, including counting one's blessings, keeping a gratitude journal, writing a gratitude letter, making a gratitude visit, and replacing ungrateful thoughts with grateful thoughts. Four studies taken together found that prayer increases the strength of gratitude (Lambert et al. 2009).

Learning from spiritual models or exemplars reduced negative religious coping and images of God as controlling and provided an avenue for learning about spirituality (Oman and Thoresen 2003; Oman et al. 2007).

Future Directions

While there is strong direction and exciting research that has emerged in the science of character, this is a field that is best described as young and developing, particularly in areas of character strength application. I have summarized some of the most recent basic and applied research on character strengths. There are a number of areas to which robust research on character strengths is needed: relationships (Does appreciation of a partner's character strengths relate to a stronger relationship?), judgment of character (What are the main variables people use to judge each of the character strengths in others?), teaching and learning (What is the impact of character strengths on classroom learning?), and connection with talents (Does alignment of signature character strengths with talents and interests lead to better performance and/or well-being than those whose signature strengths/talents/interests are not aligned?).

It is likely that each research or application point discussed in this chapter leads to further questions and research that could be conducted. For example, take the finding that some researchers have found that life satisfaction increases with degree of virtuousness (the development of character strengths); however, this increase is more apparent for the less virtuous (Ruch et al. 2007). While this is an interesting finding, it leads to many questions needing to be explored: What are the various outcomes of increasing one's character strengths? How much is enough? To what extent does one need to increase one's character strengths to buffer externalizing or addictive behaviors and mental illness? Does it cause flourishing? Does it lead to more authentic individuals, to more virtuous individuals, or both?

This is an exciting area of positive psychology. I look forward to the decade ahead for research that replicates and expands these findings, as well as research that pushes this science forward along new paths and into new territory exploring the elements of what is best in humanity.

References

Aristotle. (2000). *Nicomachean ethics* (trans: Crisp, R.). Cambridge: Cambridge University Press.

Bandura, A. (1986). *Social foundations of thought and action: A social cognitive theory*. Englewood Cliffs: Prentice Hall.

Baskin, T. W., & Enright, R. D. (2004). Intervention studies on forgiveness: A meta-analysis. *Journal of Counseling and Development, 82*, 79–80.

Baumeister, R. F., Matthew, G., DeWall, C. N., & Oaten, M. (2006). Self-regulation and personality: How interventions increase regulatory success, and how depletion moderates the effects of traits on behavior. *Journal of Personality, 74*(6), 1773–1802.

Berg, C. J., Rapoff, M. A., Snyder, C. R., & Belmont, J. M. (2007). The relationship of children's hope to pediatric asthma treatment adherence. *The Journal of Positive Psychology, 2*, 176–184.

Berkowtiz, M. W., & Gibbs, J. C. (1983). Measuring the developmental features of moral discussion. *Merrill-Palmer Quarterly, 29*, 499–410.

Biswas-Diener, R. (2006). From the equator to the North Pole: A study of character strengths. *Journal of Happiness Studies, 7*, 293–310.

Biswas-Diener, R., Kashdan, T. B., & Minhas, G. (2011). A dynamic approach to psychological strength development and intervention. *The Journal of Positive Psychology, 6*(2), 106–118.

Brdar, I., & Kashdan, T. B. (2010). Character strengths and well-being in Croatia: An empirical investigation of structure and correlates. *Journal of Research in Personality, 44*(1), 151–154.

Chory, R. M. (2007). Enhancing student perceptions of fairness: The relationship between instructor credibility and classroom justice. *Communication Education, 56*(1), 89–105.

Cooperrider, D. (2009). *The discovery and design of positive institutions*. Presented at the International Positive Psychology Association conference on June 20, 2009, PA: Philadelphia.

Cooperrider, D., & Whitney, D. (2005). *Appreciative inquiry: A positive revolution in change*. San Francisco: Berrett-Koehler.

Covington, M. V. (1999). Caring about learning: The nature and nurturing of subject-matter appreciation. *Educational Psychologist, 34*(2), 127–136.

Dahlsgaard, K., Peterson, C., & Seligman, M. E. P. (2005). Shared virtue: The convergence of valued human strengths across culture and history. *Review of General Psychology, 9*(3), 203–213.

Diessner, R., Rust, T., Solom, R., Frost, N., & Parsons, L. (2006). Beauty and hope: A moral beauty intervention. *Journal of Moral Education, 35*, 301–317.

Eisenberger, R. (1992). Learned industriousness. *Psychological Review, 99*(2), 248–267.

Emmons, R. A. (2007). *Thanks! How the new science of gratitude can make you happier*. New York: Houghton Mifflin Company.

Emmons, R. A., & McCullough, M. E. (2003). Counting blessings versus burdens: An experimental investigation of gratitude and subjective well-being in daily life. *Journal of Personality and Social Psychology, 84*, 377–389.

Finfgeld, D. (1999). Courage as a process of pushing beyond the struggle. *Qualitative Health Research, 9*, 803–814.

Flood, M., & Phillips, K. D. (2007). Creativity in older adults: A plethora of possibilities. *Issues in Mental Health Nursing, 28*, 389–411.

Fluckiger, C., & Gross Holtforth, M. G. (2008). Focusing the therapist's attention on the patient's strengths: A preliminary study to foster a mechanism of change in outpatient psychotherapy. *Journal of Clinical Psychology, 64*(7), 1–15.

Fox Eades, J. (2008). *Celebrating strengths: Building strengths-based schools*. Coventry: Capp Press.

Fredrickson, B. L., Cohn, M. A., Coffey, K. A., Pek, J., & Finkel, S. M. (2008). Open hearts build lives: Positive emotions, induced through loving-kindness meditation, build consequential personal resources. *Journal of Personality and Social Psychology, 95*(5), 1045–1062.

Froh, J. J., Sefick, W. J., & Emmons, R. A. (2008). Counting blessings in early adolescents: An experimental study of gratitude and subjective well-being. *Journal of School Psychology, 46*, 213–233.

Gable, S. L., Reis, H. T., Impett, E. A., & Asher, E. R. (2004). What do you do when things go right? The intrapersonal and interpersonal benefits of sharing positive events. *Journal of Personality and Social Psychology, 87*(2), 228–245.

Gillham, J. E., Reivich, K. J., Jaycox, L. H., & Seligman, M. E. P. (1995). Prevention of depressive symptoms in schoolchildren: Two-year follow-up. *Psychological Science, 6*, 343–351.

Gilman, R., Dooley, J., & Florell, D. (2006). Relative levels of hope and their relationship with academic and psychological indicators among adolescents. *Journal of Social and Clinical Psychology, 25*, 166–178.

Glück, J., & Baltes, P. B. (2006). Using the concept of wisdom to enhance the expression of wisdom knowledge: Not the philosopher's dream but differential effects of developmental preparedness. *Psychology and Aging, 21*, 679–690.

Hannah, S., Sweeney, P., & Lester, P. (2007). Toward a courageous mindset: The subjective act and experience of courage. *The Journal of Positive Psychology, 2*, 129–135.

Hickman, K. L., Stromme, C., & Lippman, L. G. (1998). Learned industriousness: Replication in principle. *The Journal of General Psychology, 125*(3), 213–217.

Hunter, J. P., & Csikszentmihalyi, M. (2003). The positive psychology of interested adolescents. *Journal of Youth and Adolescence, 32*(1), 27–35.

Hutcherson, C. A., Seppala, E. M., & Gross, J. J. (2008). Loving-kindness meditation increases social connection. *Emotion, 8*(5), 720–724.

King, L. A. (2001). The health benefits of writing about life goals. *Personality and Social Psychology Bulletin, 27*, 798–807.

Lambert, N. M., Fincham, F. D., Braithwaite, S. R., Graham, S. M., & Beach, S. R. H. (2009). Can prayer increase gratitude? *Psychology of Religion and Spirituality, 1*(3), 139–149.

Langer, E. (2005). *On becoming an artist: Reinventing yourself through mindful creativity*. New York: Ballantine Books.

Linley, A. (2008). *Average to A+: Realising strengths in yourself and others*. Coventry: CAPP Press.

Linley, P. A., Maltby, J., Wood, A. M., Joseph, S., Harrington, S., Peterson, C., Park, N., & Seligman, M. E. P. (2007). Character strengths in the United Kingdom: The VIA inventory of strengths. *Personality and Individual Differences, 43*, 341–351.

Linley, P. A., Nielsen, K. M., Gillett, R., & Biswas-Diener, R. (2010). Using signature strengths in pursuit of goals: Effects on goal progress, need satisfaction, and well-being, and implications for coaching psychologists. *International Coaching Psychology Review, 5*(1), 6–15.

Littman-Ovadia, H., & Davidovitch, N. (2010). Effects of congruence and character-strength deployment on work adjustment and well-being. *International Journal of Business and Social Science, 1*(3), 138–146.

Littman-Ovadia, H., & Lavy, S. (2012). Character strengths in Israel: Hebrew adaptation of the VIA Inventory of Strengths. *European Journal of Psychological Assessment, 28*(1), 41–50.

Littman-Ovadia, H., & Steger, M. (2010). Character strengths and well-being among volunteers and employees: Toward an integrative model. *The Journal of Positive Psychology, 5*(6), 419–430.

Louis, M. C. (2011). Strengths interventions in higher education: The effect of identification versus development approaches on implicit self-theory. *The Journal of Positive Psychology, 6*(3), 204–215.

Lounsbury, J. W., Fisher, L. A., Levy, J. J., & Welsh, D. P. (2009). An investigation of character strengths in relation to the academic success of college students. *Individual Differences Research, 7*(1), 52–69.

Ma, M., Kibler, J. L., Dollar, K. M., Sly, K., Samuels, D., Benford, M. W., Coleman, M., Lott, L., Patterson, K., & Wiley, F. (2008). The relationship of character strengths to sexual behaviors and related risks among African American adolescents. *International Journal of Behavioral Medicine, 15*(4), 319–327.

Macdonald, C., Bore, M., & Munro, D. (2008). Values in action scale and the big 5: An empirical indication of structure. *Journal of Research in Personality, 42*(4), 787–799.

Madden, W., Green, S., & Grant, A. M. (2011). A pilot study evaluating strengths-based coaching for primary school students: Enhancing engagement and hope. *International Coaching Psychology Review, 6*(1), 71–83.

Matthews, M. D., Eid, J., Kelly, D., Bailey, J. K. S., & Peterson, C. (2006). Character strengths and virtues of developing military leaders: An international comparison. *Military Psychology, 18*(Suppl.), S57–S68.

McCullough, M. E., Emmons, R. A., & Tsang, J. (2002). The grateful disposition: A conceptual and empirical topography. *Journal of Personality and Social Psychology, 82*, 112–127.

McCullough, M. E., Root, L. M., & Cohen, A. D. (2006). Writing about the personal benefits of a transgression facilitates forgiveness. *Journal of Consulting and Clinical Psychology, 74*, 887–897.

McGovern, T. V., & Miller, S. L. (2008). Integrating teacher behaviors with character strengths and virtues for faculty development. *Teaching of Psychology, 35*(4), 278–285.

Mitchell, J., Stanimirovic, R., Klein, B., & Vella-Brodrick, D. (2009). A randomised controlled trial of a self-guided internet intervention promoting well-being. *Computers in Human Behavior, 25*, 749–760.

Mongrain, M., & Anselmo, T. (2009). *Promise of positive interventions: Replication of Seligman et al., 2005.* Paper presented at American Psychological Association conference on August 6, 2009, Toronto.

Niemiec, R. M. (2009). *Ok, now what? Taking action.* VIA Institute. Article available at: www.viacharacter.org/www/AwareExploreApply/tabid/249/language/en-US/Default.aspx

Niemiec, R. M., & Wedding, D. (2008). *Positive psychology at the movies: Using films to build virtues and character strengths.* Cambridge, MA: Hogrefe.

Oman, D., & Thoresen, C. E. (2003). Spiritual modeling: A key to spiritual and religious growth? *The International Journal for the Psychology of Religion, 13*(3), 149–165.

Oman, D., Shapiro, S. L., Thoresen, C. E., Flinders, T., Driskill, J. D., & Plante, T. G. (2007). Learning from spiritual models and meditation: A randomized evaluation of a college course. *Pastoral Psychology, 54*, 473–493.

Onwuegbuzie, A. J. (1999). Relation of hope to self-perception. *Perceptual and Motor Skills, 88*, 535–540.

Otake, K., Shimai, S., Tanaka-Matsumi, J., Otsui, K., & Fredrickson, B. (2006). Happy people become happier through kindness: A counting kindness intervention. *Journal of Happiness Studies, 7*(3), 361–375.

Park, N., & Peterson, C. (2006a). Character strengths and happiness among young children: Content analysis of parental descriptions. *Journal of Happiness Studies, 7*, 323–341.

Park, N., & Peterson, C. (2006b). Moral competence and character strengths among adolescents: The development and validation of the values in action inventory of strengths for youth. *Journal of Adolescence, 29*, 891–905.

Park, N., & Peterson, C. (2006c). Methodological issues in positive psychology and the assessment of character strengths. In A. D. Ong & M. van Dulmen (Eds.), *Handbook of methods in positive psychology* (pp. 292–305). New York: Oxford University Press.

Park, N., & Peterson, C. (2008a). Positive psychology and character strengths: Application to strengths-based school counseling. *Professional School Counseling, 12*(2), 85–92.

Park, N., & Peterson, C. (2008b). The cultivation of character strengths. In M. Ferrari & G. Poworowski (Eds.), *Teaching for wisdom* (pp. 57–75). Mahwah: Erlbaum.

Park, N., & Peterson, C. (2009a). Character strengths: Research and practice. *Journal of College and Character, 10*(4), np.

Park, N., & Peterson, C. (2009b). Strengths of character in schools. In R. Gilman, E. S. Huebner, & M. J. Furlong (Eds.), *Handbook of positive psychology in schools* (pp. 65–76). New York: Routledge.

Park, N., Peterson, C., & Seligman, M. E. P. (2004). Strengths of character and well-being. *Journal of Social and Clinical Psychology, 23*, 603–619.

Park, N., Peterson, C., & Seligman, M. E. P. (2006). Character strengths in fifty-four nations and the fifty US states. *The Journal of Positive Psychology, 1*(3), 118–129.

Park, N., Peterson, C., & Ruch, W. (2009). Orientations to happiness and life satisfaction in twenty-seven nations. *The Journal of Positive Psychology, 4*(4), 273–279.

Peterson, C., & Park, N. (2009). Classifying and measuring strengths of character. In S. J. Lopez & C. R. Snyder (Eds.), *Oxford handbook of positive psychology* (2nd ed., pp. 25–33). New York: Oxford University Press.

Peterson, T. D., & Peterson, E. W. (2008). Stemming the tide of law student depression: What law schools need to learn from the science of positive psychology. *Yale Journal of Health Policy, Law, and Ethics, 9*(2): 357–434. Available at: http://ssrn.com/abstract=1277303

Peterson, C., & Seligman, M. E. P. (2003). Character strengths before and after September 11. *Psychological Science, 14*, 381–384.

Peterson, C., & Seligman, M. E. P. (2004). *Character strengths and virtues: A handbook and classification*. New York: Oxford University Press/Washington, DC: American Psychological Association.

Peterson, C., Park, N., & Seligman, M. E. P. (2006). Greater strengths of character and recovery from illness. *The Journal of Positive Psychology, 1*(1), 17–26.

Peterson, C., Ruch, W., Beerman, U., Park, N., & Seligman, M. E. P. (2007). Strengths of character, orientations to happiness, and life satisfaction. *The Journal of Positive Psychology, 2*, 149–156.

Peterson, C., Park, N., Pole, N., D'Andrea, W., & Seligman, M. E. P. (2008). Strengths of character and posttraumatic growth. *Journal of Traumatic Stress, 21*, 214–217.

Peterson, C., Park, N., Hall, N., & Seligman, M. E. P. (2009). Zest and work. *Journal of Organizational Behavior, 30*, 161–172.

Pury, C. (2008). Can courage be learned? In S. J. Lopez (Ed.), *Positive psychology: Exploring human strengths* (pp. 109–130). Westport: Praeger.

Ruch, W., Huber, A., Beermann, U., & Proyer, R. T. (2007). Character strengths as predictors of the "good life" in Austria, Germany and Switzerland. In Romanian Academy, "George Barit" Institute of History, Department of Social Research (Ed.), *Studies and researches in social sciences* (Vol. 16) (pp. 123–131). Cluj-Napoca: Argonaut Press.

Ruch, W., Proyer, R. T., Harzer, C., Park, N., Peterson, C., & Seligman, M. E. P. (2010). Values in action inventory of strengths (VIA-IS): Adaptation and validation of the German version and the development of a peer-rating form. *Journal of Individual Differences, 31*(3), 138–149.

Rust, T., Diessner, R., & Reade, L. (2009). Strengths only or strengths and relative weaknesses? A preliminary study. *Journal of Psychology, 143*(5), 465–476.

Schwartz, B., & Sharpe, K. E. (2006). Practical wisdom: Aristotle meets positive psychology. *Journal of Happiness Studies, 7*, 377–395.

Scott, G., Leritz, L. E., & Mumford, M. D. (2004). The effectiveness of creativity training: A quantitative review. *Creativity Research Journal, 16*(4), 361–388.

Seligman, M. E. P. (2002). *Authentic happiness*. New York: Free Press.

Seligman, M. E. P., & Csikszentmihalyi, M. (2000). Positive psychology: An introduction. *American Psychologist, 55*, 5–14.

Seligman, M. E. P., Steen, T. A., Park, N., & Peterson, C. (2005). Positive psychology progress: Empirical validation of interventions. *American Psychologist, 60*, 410–421.

Seligman, M. E. P., Rashid, T., & Parks, A. (2006). Positive psychotherapy. *American Psychologist, 61*, 774–778.

Sheldon, K. M., & Lyubomirsky, S. (2006). How to increase and sustain positive emotion: The effects of expressing gratitude and visualizing best possible selves. *The Journal of Positive Psychology, 1*, 73–82.

Shimai, S., Otake, K., Park, N., Peterson, C., & Seligman, M. E. P. (2006). Convergence of character strengths in American and Japanese young adults. *Journal of Happiness Studies, 7*, 311–322.

Shryack, J., Steger, M. F., Krueger, R. F., & Kallie, C. S. (2010). The Structure of virtue: An empirical investigation of the dimensionality of the virtues in action inventory of strengths. *Personality and Individual Differences, 48*, 714–719.

Singh, K., & Choubisa, R. (2010). Empirical validation of values in action-inventory of strengths (VIA-IS) in Indian context. *Psychological Studies, 55*(2), 151–158.

Staats, S., Hupp, J. M., & Hagley, A. M. (2008). Honesty and heroes: A positive psychology view of heroism and academic honesty. *The Journal of Psychology, 142*(4), 357–372.

Steger, M. F., Hicks, B., Kashdan, T. B., Krueger, R. F., & Bouchard, T. J., Jr. (2007). Genetic and environmental influences on the positive traits of the values in action classification, and biometric covariance with normal personality. *Journal of Research in Personality, 41*, 524–539.

Sumner-Armstrong, C., Newcombe, P., & Martin, R. (2008). A qualitative investigation into leader behavioural flexibility. *The Journal of Management Development, 27*(8), 843–857.

Sweeney, P., Hannah, S. T., Park, N., Peterson, C., Matthews, M., & Brazil, D. (2009). *Character strengths, adaptation, and trust*. Paper presented at the International Positive Psychology Association conference on June 19, 2009, PA: Philadelphia.

Tedeschi, R. G., & Calhoun, L. G. (1995). *Trauma and transformation: Growing in the aftermath of suffering*. Thousand Oaks, CA: Sage.

Tetlock, P. E. (1986). A value pluralism model of ideological reasoning. *Journal of Personality and Social Psychology, 50*, 819–827.

Vella-Brodrick, D. A., Park, N., & Peterson, C. (2009). Three ways to be happy: Pleasure, engagement, and meaning. Findings from Australian and US samples. *Social Indicators Research, 90*, 165–179.

Wade, N. G., Worthington, E. L., & Meyer, J. E. (2005). But do they work? A meta-analysis of group interventions to promote forgiveness. In E. L. Worthington (Ed.), *Handbook of forgiveness* (pp. 423–439). New York: Routledge.

West, B. J., Patera, J. L., & Carsten, M. K. (2009). Team level positivity: Investigating positive psychological capacities and team level outcomes. *Journal of Organizational Behavior, 30*, 249–267.

Wong, Y. J. (2006). Strength-centered therapy: A social constructionist, virtues-based psychotherapy. *Psychotherapy: Theory, Research, Practice, Training, 43*(2), 133–146.

Chapter 3
Addressing Current Challenges in Cross-Cultural Measurement of Well-Being: The Pemberton Happiness Index

Carmelo Vazquez and Gonzalo Hervas

Challenges in Current Cross-Cultural Research

The study of culture provides a fascinating window through which we can detect systematic factors (e.g., wealth, social inequalities, values, and social norms) associated with well-being. Several in-depth reviews describe the main findings on this issue (e.g., Diener et al. 2003; Diener and Suh 2000; Mesquita and Leu 2007; Suh and Koo 2008; Morrison et al. 2011; Tov and Diener 2007). Yet, comparing nations or cultures with respect to an outcome such as happiness or well-being is problematic as there are methodological and conceptual issues that must be taken into account.

In this chapter, we focus on three specific challenges that are very pertinent to cross-cultural research on well-being and that have not received enough attention.[1] The first two issues tackle *what* and *how* to measure. That is, when we measure well-being in different nations and cultures, what are we measuring and what exactly should we measure? Once we decide what to measure, it is important to be aware that the methods we use may significantly affect the type of information we actually gather. The third issue has to do with the need for solid but brief indicators that are able to capture the complexity of well-being.

---

[1] A potential problem in cross-cultural research that we do not discuss here is the differential pattern of response styles among countries. For example, Vittersø et al. (2005) found that Norwegians and Greenlanders did not differ in their mean scores on a life satisfaction scale, but latent trait analyses showed that Greenlanders tended to answer all items of the questionnaire more randomly and more extremely. Kapteyn et al. (2010) described a similar effect when comparing life satisfaction estimations of American and Dutch participants: The Dutch were more avoidant of making extreme negative or positive evaluations. Other issues reviewed in the literature (e.g., order of items, item functioning, or scale numbers), although important independently (e.g., Deaton 2011), do not seem to substantially affect cross-cultural comparisons (see Oishi 2010).

C. Vazquez (✉) • G. Hervas
Department of Clinical Psychology, School of Psychology,
Complutense University, 28223, Madrid, Spain
e-mail: cvazquez@psi.ucm.es; ghervas@psi.ucm.es

H.H. Knoop and A. Delle Fave (eds.), *Well-Being and Cultures: Perspectives from Positive Psychology*, Cross-Cultural Advancements in Positive Psychology 3, DOI 10.1007/978-94-007-4611-4_3, © Springer Science+Business Media Dordrecht 2013

First Challenge: What to Measure

When attempting to compare well-being across cultures, we must clarify the concept of well-being, which is implicitly or explicitly addressed by the measures used. There is now consensus in this field of research that subjective well-being (SWB) is composed of two components: life satisfaction and affect balance (a presence of positive emotions alongside a low presence of negative emotions) (Diener 1984). One important difference between these two components is that judgments of life satisfaction are more abstract and cognitive in nature than evaluations of emotional state (Lucas et al. 1996). The distinction between cognitive and emotional components of well-being is highly relevant to cross-cultural research as it has been shown that life satisfaction judgments are global estimations of well-being and, therefore, are more dependent on cultural norms and values than specific assessments (Diener et al. 2010).

When comparing results on well-being among different countries, one should consider the type of components being evaluated. For example, some countries present relatively high scores on measures of life satisfaction but less high on positive affect and vice versa: Laos ranks very high on enjoyment but comes in at 132nd on more global measures of life satisfaction (cit. Oishi 2010). Furthermore, these two well-being components correlate differentially depending on societal and personal variables. For instance, whereas life satisfaction seems closely linked to personal achievements and societal circumstances (e.g., a personal education or a nation's wealth) (Diener et al. 2009; Kahneman et al. 2006), respondents' emotions (e.g., joy or sadness) are more linked to daily circumstances and events (Diener et al. 2010). It is crucial to be informed of these different facets of SWB to adequately interpret cross-cultural data.[2] The mere consideration of these two components makes it rather pointless to establish "ranks" of nations on well-being as these ranks depend on indicators used.

To increase the complexity, cultural factors also influence how people report different types of affect. In a study of momentary assessment of affect with samples of students from different cultures, Scollon et al. (2004) found greater cross-cultural differences in positive emotions than in negative emotions. Consistent with this finding, a meta-analysis of cross-cultural variation in emotions revealed more unexplained variance in assessments of positive compared to negative emotions (Van Hemert et al. 2007). In their review on this topic, Scollon et al. (2011) examined different hypotheses that may explain these differences. First, positive emotions are rated as more desirable than negative ones in Western but not Asian cultures (Eid and Diener 2001); on the other hand, a large percentage of respondents in countries like China rated all negative emotions as desirable responses, but this was not the case in Western countries (i.e., Australia and the USA). Second, ratings of desirability

---

[2] Furthermore, people can judge life satisfaction from a general perspective or through specific domains of satisfaction (e.g., with friends, family, education, neighborhood, or work) which may lead to different results (Diener et al. 2000).

correlate positively with the display of particular emotions (Eid and Diener 2001). Thus, cultural metacognition about the value of positive and negative emotions can contribute to regulate the expression of these emotions and the feelings and valuations associated with them.

Nevertheless, well-being is not limited to the exploration of SWB. Well-being concerns not only an optimal experience, which is fairly encompassed by the concept of SWB, but also eudaemonia or optimal psychological functioning (Ryan and Deci 2001). There have been recent discussions on whether eudaemonic variables are necessary to assess well-being. Some authors argue that SWB is related to both hedonic and eudaemonic well-being, and that evaluating other variables with SWB makes it difficult to differentiate predictors and outcomes of well-being (Kashdan et al. 2008). In contrast, authors of the eudaemonic tradition argue that any well-being measure without a eudaemonic component would be incomplete (Keyes and Annas 2009; Ryan and Huta 2009). In support of the latter assertion, some people can feel happy and report experiencing happiness yet lack other relevant features that characterize a psychologically healthy person (Ryan and Huta 2009). Individuals skilled at self-deception or with psychological disorders (i.e., mania), for example, could present a high level of SWB but exhibit a low level of daily functioning and self-realization at the same time.

An emphasis on eudaemonic components of well-being does not mean that SWB is a marginal component of a good life. On the contrary, as some authors have pointed out (Kashdan et al. 2008), life satisfaction and positive affect do not simply measure hedonic well-being. Research has demonstrated that these hedonic measures are also strongly associated with eudaemonic experiences (e.g., Ryan and Huta 2009; Waterman 2008) and optimal functioning (Lyubomirsky et al. 2005). Thus, an integrative assessment of well-being requires assessing both affect (including judgment of the global quality of one's own life) and overall functioning (Delle Fave and Bassi 2009; Keyes and Annas 2009; Tamir and Gross 2011).

Even after incorporating eudaemonic aspects, there is still one component lacking to complete the picture of well-being. Beyond the distinction between hedonic and eudaemonic well-being, some authors have expanded this individualistic perspective by including societal features related to personal feelings of well-being. In his influential proposal on optimal functioning and mental health, Keyes (1998) noted that "individuals remain embedded in social structures and communities, and face countless social tasks and challenges" (p. 122). According to this author, the appraisal of one's circumstances and functioning in society, what he calls "social well-being," is also necessary for integrative models of well-being.

Thus, the question is not what single variable we should assess but what components we should include in a multifaceted assessment of well-being. Measuring the latent construct of well-being implies the assessment of a wide range of elements such as life satisfaction, affect, positive functioning, and social well-being.

Beyond these arguments, there is another reason; it is important to include several facets when measuring well-being. Oishi (2010) recently discussed whether concepts like "happiness" or "well-being" are exactly equivalent in different languages and cultures. Although it seems plausible that most people in any culture are able to assess their own emotional experiences and quality of life, it is likely that the connotations of the labels used to describe these emotions and judgments are not identical to those in published research (mostly lead by Western researchers). In fact, some basic emotions have no identifiable labels in certain languages (Russell 1991). For example, when asked to describe the meaning of "well-being," American students typically bring up feelings of "excitement" or heightened arousal, whereas Chinese students mention feelings of "calm" or equilibrium (Lu and Gilmour 2004). Furthermore, words such as "happiness" are spontaneously associated with positive words by American college students, whereas their Japanese counterparts provide associations with both positive and negative words. In a recent study using a lexical probabilistic procedure with university samples from different countries (Chile, Colombia, Germany, Palestine, and the USA), Vargas (2010) found that the idea that "happiness" is difficult to obtain or transitory is negatively associated with self-reported life satisfaction in students from Spain but shows no significant association with life satisfaction in students from the USA. Interestingly, the concept of "happiness" can vary not only across space (i.e., nations or cultures) but also time. As Oishi (2010) points out, words such as "happiness" have undergone significant changes in their official definition (e.g., in standard dictionaries) and use in the last century.[3]

Thus, differences on the concept of happiness or well-being among countries constitute another reason to incorporate scales or items that do not explicitly include these culturally unclear ideas into standard well-being or happiness measures.

Second Challenge: How to Measure

There are many different measures available for each component of well-being addressed in the previous pages. Most of these measures have been subjected to scrupulous psychometric analyses, and some have also been validated in different countries and languages (see a review of measures in Lopez and Snyder 2003; Eid 2008).

Measures of well-being may differ not only in their content (e.g., hedonic and eudaemonic components) and format (e.g., open-ended questions, interviews, or questionnaires)[4] but also with regard to time frame. In the vast majority of available

---

[3] According to his review, in many countries, there has been a secular shift in the meaning of "happiness" from an emphasis on "lucky and fortunate conditions" to inner feeling states. Incidentally, Diener (2000) found that in countries where "happiness" is mainly used to define satisfaction of one's goals and desires (e.g., Spain or Italy), happiness is seen as more desirable than in countries or regions where happiness is defined in terms of luck (e.g., East Asia, France, Germany, and Russia).

[4] Most current measures of well-being are based on self-reports, even though self-reports of emotional states can be vulnerable to self-presentation biases, memory biases, and the ability to perceive and label emotions. Some authors have proposed alternative procedures based on reaction time to probe stimulus or in experimental measures to assess implicit beliefs (e.g., Diaz et al. 2009).

measures, participants are asked to report their well-being on a scale within a given temporal framework (e.g., past week, past month, or in general). As such, most data researchers that have gathered on well-being in the last fruitful decades have focused on retrospective accounts of well-being (i.e., remembered well-being) (Kahneman and Krueger 2006). These measures have been the basis for current theories of well-being, and there is strong evidence that, beyond some methodological issues (e.g., linguistic equivalence of terms), these measures effectively reflect emotional states.

Although retrospective judgments are standard for obtaining significant personal information and have been extensively used in most areas of psychology, there is also evidence that these judgments are affected by a number of cognitive and motivational factors (Kahneman 1999). Interestingly, these factors may affect different cultures in idiosyncratic ways. A number of studies have demonstrated that the method used to assess psychological variables may in fact be a source of significant cross-cultural differences in and of itself.

For example, Yamaguchi et al. (2007) found that American students had significantly higher scores than Japanese students in explicit measures of self-esteem (i.e., a standard questionnaire) as many other studies have found, but these differences disappeared when using an implicit measure that does not require self-report evaluations (e.g., the Implicit Association Test; see footnote #4).

More directly related to our field, Oishi (2002) compared well-being reports of Asian and European Americans and found that although European Americans reported a higher degree of well-being than Asians in retrospective global reports (i.e., remembered well-being), there were no cultural differences in current well-being assessed by a daily diary or using an online measure. In this study, the author used Experience Sampling Methodology (ESM), which involves asking respondents to report what they are currently doing and/or feeling.[5] Oishi asked participants to estimate their daily satisfaction level for seven consecutive days and to also respond to random signals on how happy they felt at that moment (ESM) during the same period. Results showed that although Asian Americans and European Americans did not differ in their average satisfaction level, recorded daily in their diaries, European Americans expressed higher satisfaction than Asian Americans in a global retrospective judgment of the week. The same pattern of results was found for the ESM part of the study: Both samples did not differ in the proportion of random moments they said they were happy, but Asian Americans reported having had less moments of happiness than European Americans when asked to retrospectively estimate the frequency of happy moments they had in the week of the data collection.

Similar memory biases have been found in other studies (Oishi and Diener 2003; Wirtz et al. 2003). For instance, Wirtz et al. (2003) found no differences in average daily satisfaction level over 21 days in European Americans, Asian Americans,

---

[5] Although there are several types of ESM procedures (see Scollon et al. 2003), this approach has provided valuable online data, which are not subject to cognitive biases linked to retrospective accounts.

Japanese, and Koreans, but European Americans reported higher total scores than Asian Americans on the Satisfaction with Life Scale (SWLS; Diener et al. 1985). An ESM study by Scollon et al. (2004) presented an exception when the authors found significant differences among Hispanic American, European American, Japanese, and Indian participants in experienced positive emotions at random moments but did not find memory biases in recalling the frequency of these moments.

Along these lines, another artificial source of variance in cross-cultural well-being is tied to the cognitive processes associated with retrospective judgments. When participants from different nations are asked about their life satisfaction or happiness, they may use different heuristics or cognitive strategies to arrive at a conclusion. There is increasing evidence that these cognitive processes are rather complex and are moderated by cultural norms and the perceived importance of emotions. In a study involving five countries, Schimmack et al. (2002) found that people in individualistic nations seem to depend more on their own current emotional states to make inferences on their life satisfaction (i.e., correlations of emotions and life satisfaction were stronger in individualistic nations than in collectivistic ones). Thus, people seem to judge their life satisfaction based, at least in part, on how they value their emotions, and this, in turn, is affected by cultural values (see Scollon et al. 2011).

Although the results are not entirely consistent, there is rather reliable initial evidence suggesting that cross-cultural differences in well-being are, to some extent, related to the use of different memory strategies or heuristics to make global judgments of life satisfaction or happiness.

Importantly, retrospective does not necessarily mean more biased or less reliable. Research has demonstrated that both retrospective and online measures can be used separately to predict different outcomes (Scollon et al. 2003). Despite their apparent generality, global reports covering extended periods of time can be useful in predicting outcomes and behavioral choices. For example, Wirtz et al. (2003) investigated the differential ability of online experiences, retrospective recall, and expectation to determine future behavior. In their study, vacationing students completed self-reports measuring expectations of pleasure, online reports of pleasure, and retrospective recall of pleasure. Results indicated that only retrospective recall significantly predicted the desire to take a similar vacation in the future. Thus, both types of approaches should be considered necessary and complementary.

Unfortunately, alternative methodologies to assess well-being, such as the ESM or DRM, are very costly and/or time consuming when it comes to generalized use in cross-cultural research. A typical ESM study lasts 1–2 weeks with 2–12 daily signals (Reis and Gable 2000) and can be very disruptive of daily activities. Although DRM studies are not as expensive as ESM studies, they may take up to 1 h for each participant to obtain a detailed description of what happened in the last 24 h. The Gallup International survey has adopted a more modest strategy where measurement of affect is based on whether respondents have experienced a number of positive feelings (i.e., enjoyment and smiling/laughter) or negative feelings (i.e., sadness, anger, worry, and depression) over the past 24 h. Respondents are asked to remember if they experienced these feelings (yes/no responses), and an Affect Balance score is calculated by averaging both scores and subtracting positive from negative experiences (Diener et al. 2010). Nevertheless, we should not forget that none of these methodologies are free of issues that affect all measures of well-being (e.g., number use, item functioning, cultural norms, response biases, and self-presentation biases) (Schwarz 1999).

In sum, apart from the *what, how* we measure well-being is also very relevant to ensure a sound exploration of cross-cultural differences in well-being. These differences may depend on the type of component we are measuring (e.g., satisfaction with life vs. emotional balance) and also on the measurement strategy used (e.g., retrospective vs. online).

Third Challenge: The Search for Efficient Measures

Results showing differences in well-being among countries have provided hints on how, for example, societal variables may affect individuals' well-being (e.g., Veenhoven 2000; Oishi and Schimmack 2010; Schimmack et al. 2005). To reach solid conclusions, cross-cultural studies need large samples of participants. Unfortunately, the larger the sample, the more difficult it becomes to conduct long interviews or implement well-validated questionnaires aimed at measuring specific facets of well-being. The more direct way to overcome this problem is with short but reliable and comprehensive measures of well-being. Consequently, the development of cost-efficient alternative methods that are relatively immune to culture-based biases is an important challenge for current research on well-being.

Most national and international surveys on well-being with large samples have relied on single items covering global satisfaction or happiness. This approach, however limited, has produced comparable and meaningful data (Oswald and Wu 2010; Veenhoven 2007, 2009), and these relatively simple indices have been linked to outcomes such as stronger social relationships and marital satisfaction (Diener and Seligman 2002), productivity (Lyubomirsky et al. 2005), physical and mental health (Vázquez et al. 2009, 2011), and even longevity (Diener and Chan 2011; Xu and Roberts 2010).

The time frame used to explore well-being is pertinent when using simple questions. When the time frame is wide (e.g., "All things considered, how satisfied are you with life as a whole these days?" or "Taking all things together, how would you say things are these days?: 1 – very happy, 2 – quite happy, 3 – not very happy, or 4 – not at all happy?"),[6] it is more likely that a general knowledge of oneself influences answers, whereas what people actually did or felt may influence answers if the time frame is more narrow (e.g., "How did you feel yesterday?"). Although there is little direct evidence of this assertion, a study by Scollon et al. (2009) seems to support this argument. In their study, participants completed daily and retrospective

---

[6] These questions are included in the World Values Survey.

measures of well-being for a 1-week period. The results demonstrated that participants' notion of "ideal well-being," which is shaped by culturally created values and
expectations, correlated more highly with retrospective measures than with momentary measures of well-being. Thus, it is important to keep in mind that the type of
general questions typically illustrating cross-national differences, such as those in
the World Database of Happiness (Veenhoven 2011), can shape respondents'
answers as a function of their format.

Another interesting methodological issue concerns the distribution of scores each
scale yields. Many international comparisons of well-being are based on single items
that tap into the construct of global satisfaction with life. Yet interestingly, not all
items offer the same score distribution despite their apparent conceptual similarity.
For example, the Gallup study used two items to assess global perceptions of one's
own life: a measure of satisfaction with life using a scale from 0 (*dissatisfied*) to 10
(*satisfied*) and Cantril's Ladder Scale (Cantril 1965), which asks respondents to evaluate their lives on a scale from 0 (*worst possible*) to 10 (*best possible*). Respondents are
required to select the step on the ladder where they believe they stand at the present
time. Notably, whereas the satisfaction-with-life item is negatively skewed (i.e., the
mean is well above 5, and there are many more individuals rating their lives above the
central point than below it; see also Cummins and Nistico 2002), the Cantril's Ladder
distribution is nearly normally distributed (see Helliwell and Barrington-Leigh 2010).

The affective component of well-being has also been covered in international
studies such as the World Values Survey (http://www.worldvaluessurvey.org) where
"happiness" is measured with one item: "Taking all things together, would you say
you are?" (1 Very happy; 2 Quite happy; 3 Not very happy; 4 Not at all happy) – see
above. The Gallup International survey, as previously described, measures affect by
counting the number of positive or negative feelings experienced during the past 24 h.

Thus, there are several simple ways to measure components of SWB that have
served to make sound cross-national comparisons, although in general, these studies
have mostly ignored other facets of well-being (e.g., eudaemonic or social well-
being) and have used a limited range of methods; for instance, no large-scale international study has implemented diaries or online methodologies despite the interest
in these types of approaches from a cross-cultural perspective.

Recently, various brief measures have been developed that tap into other aspects of
the multifaceted well-being construct. As an example, Diener and his team designed
the Flourishing Scale (FS; Diener et al. 2009) "to measure social–psychological prosperity, [and] to complement existing measures of subjective well-being" (p. 144). The
FS is an eight-item scale covering aspects of social capital, flow, social relationships,
and a general sense of psychological prosperity (e.g., "I am a good person and live a
good life," "I lead a purposeful and meaningful life," and "People respect me"). This
new scale was aimed at measuring "flourishing" through a single index.

Another interesting new instrument is the Warwick-Edinburgh Mental Well-
Being Scale (WEMWBS; Tennant et al. 2007), designed primarily for use in large-
scale public policy analyses. This scale comprises 14 positively phrased statements
covering both hedonic and eudaemonic aspects of positive mental health, including
positive affect, satisfying interpersonal relationships, and positive functioning.

Participants are provided with a general framework to make retrospective judgments on these aspects of well-being: "In the last two weeks, I've been feeling… (cheerful, good about myself, relaxed, useful, interested in other people, etc.)." The authors also recently published a seven-item version of the scale that seems to better fit a unidimensional structure of positive mental health (Stewart-Brown et al. 2009).

These two measures have two important features. First, they are short, making them apt for large-scale studies, and second, they include different components of well-being such as hedonic and/or eudaemonic constructs. However, they fail to include important components such as social well-being (both WEMWBS and FS), global life satisfaction (WEMWBS), and autonomy (FS). Thus, although there have been important advances in this field of measurement, the development of short and comprehensive indices of well-being remains a challenge for the future.

The Pemberton Happiness Index: Measuring Remembered and Experienced Well-Being

To respond to these challenges, we recently developed and validated a brief instrument to measure integrative well-being (Hervas and Vazquez 2012). Our objective was to create a brief scale that (a) covered different domains of well-being (i.e., general, hedonic, eudemonic, and social), (b) tapped into different approaches through which well-being is assessed (i.e., remembered and experienced well-being), and (c) was validated for a variety of languages (and countries) from its inception.

As distinctive characteristics of the scale's construction process, the validation was conducted simultaneously in seven languages (English, German, Japanese, Russian, Spanish, Swedish, and Turkish) through the Computer-Assisted Web Interviewing (CAWI) technique with a relatively high number of participants ($N=4,052$).

Participants were recruited from research panels (i.e., groups of people that agree to regularly participate in social surveys) of Millward Brown, an international survey company with branches in each participating country. For the initial study, we selected nine countries from diverse linguistic, religious, and cultural backgrounds.

All participants responded to an initial pool of items covering different facets of well-being. These items were divided into two main areas: remembered well-being and experienced well-being.

1. *Remembered Well-Being.* We generated items that had similar content to those included in well-known validated measures of well-being. An initial pool of 21 items was created to assess four domains of remembered well-being (i.e., general, eudaemonic, hedonic, and social well-being). Each domain or subdomain (eudaemonic well-being has six subdomains, and hedonic well-being has two subdomains) consisted of at least two items. Participants were asked to rate each

of the 21 statements using a scale from 0 (*fully disagree*) to 10 (*fully agree*). Item translation followed standard translation and back-translation procedures.

(a) *General Well-Being.* We included two items related to global satisfaction with life and one item of vitality as it is closely associated with eudaemonic functioning (e.g., Ryan and Frederick 1997).
(b) *Eudaemonic Well-Being.* Items covering optimal psychological functioning were derived from Ryff's psychological well-being model (Ryff 1989; Ryff and Keyes 1995). We put together a set of 12 items addressing the following subdomains equivalent to Ryff's six areas of psychological well-being: life meaning, self-acceptance, personal growth, relatedness, perceived control, and autonomy.
(c) *Hedonic Well-Being.* Affective state was assessed with items reflecting the frequency of positive and negative affect in daily life with two items for each affect type.
(d) *Social Well-Being.* Although there are several components of social well-being (see Keyes 1998; Keyes et al. 2002), we selected two items that tap into the global feeling of living in a society that promotes optimal psychological functioning (i.e., social actualization).

2. *Experienced Well-Being.* As previously mentioned, it is a challenge to create reliable and efficient measures of experienced well-being. Following a strategy similar to that of the Gallup-Healthways Well-Being Index (Harter and Gurley 2008), which in turn was based on the DRM (Kahneman et al. 2004), we generated a list of 16 items related to specific experiences that may have happened the day before in any of the countries. Thus, participants were presented with eight common positive events (e.g., "I did something fun with someone") and eight negative ones (e.g., "Things happened that made me really angry") that can be experienced by virtually anyone on a given day in different cultures. Participants were simply asked to state whether or not any of these events occurred the day before.

In an effort to establish a solid instrument, aside from this initial pool of 37 items specifically generated for our scale (21 related to remembered well-being and 16 related to experienced well-being), participants also responded to a series of well-known instruments assessing the areas of well-being covered by the items. These measures, all included in the CAWI system, were used as criteria for the final selection of items for our new scale. We chose convergent validity as the main criterion, so selected items were those that showed the highest mean correlations with their respective validation measures across countries. Thus, rather than validating an overall score of the new proposed scale, we implemented an empirically based process to select the items that would be included in the final scale, choosing items that presented the highest correlations with the scales or subscales that covered the relevant content of well-being. For example, to tap into the facet of positive affect, we selected the item demonstrating the highest correlation with the positive affect subscale from the Positive and Negative Affect Schedule (PANAS; Watson et al. 1988).

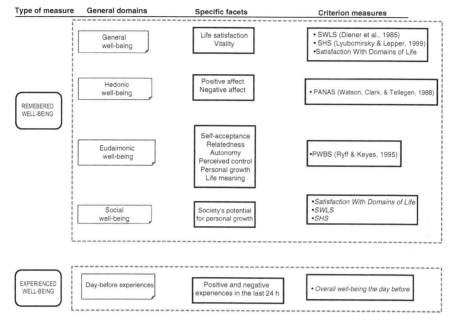

Fig. 3.1 Summary of the components of remembered and experienced well-being included in the PHI. The *second column* details the components, the *third column* presents the facets of our measure, and the *fourth column* illustrates the measures used as criteria to validate each specific facet

We included the SWLS (Diener et al. 1985), the Subjective Happiness Scale (SHS; Lyubomirsky and Lepper 1999), Satisfaction with Domains of Life (SWDL; participants rated their satisfaction with 12 domains of life selected from Cummins 2006; Diener et al. 1985; and Huebner et al. 1999), and the Psychological Well-Being Scales (SPWB; Ryff and Keyes 1995) to validate the items measuring eudaemonic well-being; the PANAS (Watson et al. 1988) to validate the items associated with hedonic well-being; and the SWDL item that assesses satisfaction with one's own country, as well as total scores from the SWLS and SHS to validate the items related to global social well-being (see Fig. 3.1).

To validate our measure of experienced well-being (i.e., experiences that occurred the day before), we included a question aimed at assessing the participant's overall well-being experienced the day before (i.e., "How did you feel yesterday?") rated on a Likert scale from 0 (*very badly*) to 4 (*great*).[7]

Correlations between each of the 21 initial remembered well-being items and their respective comparison scales were calculated for each country to reach a

---

[7] Chi-square analyses were conducted between each item and the criterion (i.e., overall satisfaction with the day before). Items that showed the highest overall mean eta-squared values were selected for inclusion in the final scale.

Table 3.1 Domains and subdomains of the Pemberton Happiness Index and their corresponding items

Domains and subdomains	Item content
Remembered well-being	
General well-being	I am very satisfied with my life
	I have the energy to accomplish my daily tasks
Eudaemonic well-being	
Life meaning	I think my life is useful and worthwhile
Self-acceptance	I am satisfied with myself
Personal growth	My life is full of learning experiences and challenges that make me grow
Relatedness	I feel very connected to the people around me
Perceived control	I feel able to solve the majority of my daily problems
Autonomy	I think that I can be myself on the important things
Hedonic well-being	
Positive affect	I enjoy a lot of little things every day
Negative affect	I have a lot of bad moments in my daily life
Social well-being	I think that I live in a society that lets me fully realize my potential
Experienced well-being	
Positive experiences	Something I did made me proud
	I did something fun with someone
	I did something I really enjoy doing
	I learned something interesting
	I gave myself a treat
Negative experiences	At times, I felt overwhelmed
	I was bored for a lot of the time
	I was worried about personal matters
	Things happened that made me really angry
	I felt disrespected by someone

final scale with the highest possible concurrent validity for all countries. Items that presented the highest overall mean correlations with their corresponding criteria were chosen to be included in the final scale. The final items are presented in Table 3.1.

Scoring Remembered and Experienced Well-Being in the PHI

The Pemberton Happiness Index (PHI) was designed as a brief measure of overall well-being that includes both remembered *and* experienced well-being. Although data for these two types of well-being can be separately obtained in the PHI, a procedure was designed to provide a combined well-being index. To obtain this overall index, the number of positive experiences is added to the number of absences of negative experiences (i.e., each positive experience of the day before is counted as "1," and the sum of absences of negative experiences is added to this partial score).

With this procedure, a single overall score of experienced well-being can be calculated, ranging from 0 to 10 similarly to the previous items. Other researchers have used this method in the past to reach a single score based on positive and negative experiences of the day before (e.g., Diener et al. 2010).

Thus, the PHI can be utilized both as a measure of separate retrospective and remembered components and as a single indicator of well-being: (a) an 11-item measure that includes general, eudaemonic, hedonic, and social well-being rated on a scale from 0 to 10 and (b) a single score that results from the combination of positive and negative experiences from the day before, also on a scale from 0 to 10.

Table 3.1 shows the final items empirically selected for the PHI. It contains 11 items related to different domains of remembered well-being (i.e., general, eudaemonic, hedonic, and social well-being) and 10 items related to experienced well-being, which can be transformed into a single well-being index using the same scale as the other 11 items.

Psychometric Properties of the PHI

Initial psychometric data of the PHI are encouraging (Hervas and Vazquez 2012). In the preliminary validation study, the internal consistency of the scales (in both the 11-item version and 11 + 1-item version) was above .89 in all countries with the exception of the Turkey sample (Cronbach's alpha from .82 to .83). In the same study, the internal consistency values for the SWLS (Diener et al. 1985), although high (from .83 to .91), were generally lower than for the PHI. Thus, the PHI compares favorably with standard measures of life satisfaction, one of the main components of SWB.

Using a series of separate regression analyses, we determined the PHI's incremental validity when matched with recognized well-being scales. Sleep quality and perceived health, which often represent well-being (Hervas and Vazquez 2012), were implemented as criteria. Our results demonstrated that the PHI predicted sleep quality better than the SHS ($\Delta R^2 = .029$, $p < .001$), SWLS ($\Delta R^2 = .056$, $p < .001$), SPWB ($\Delta R^2 = .052$, $p < .001$), and PANAS ($\Delta R^2 = .040$, $p < .001$). The PHI also outperformed the SHS ($\Delta R^2 = .042$, $p < .001$), SWLS ($\Delta R^2 = .088$, $p < .001$), SPWB ($\Delta R^2 = .052$, $p < .001$), and PANAS ($\Delta R^2 = .051$, $p < .001$) in predicting perceived health.

Remembered Versus Experienced Well-Being

Discrepancies between remembered and experienced well-being are very intriguing. It is remarkable that in this study, participants from Japan presented significantly lower scores in both remembered and experienced well-being. More importantly, Japan is the only country in which scores on remembered well-being were significantly lower than scores on experienced well-being when using comparable metrics (Hervas and Vazquez 2010; see Fig. 3.2). This result is congruent with previous research conducted by Oishi (2002) who found that European Americans

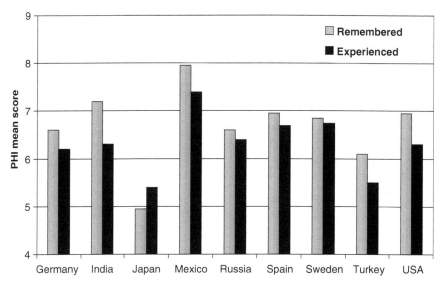

Fig. 3.2 A comparison of remembered and experienced well-being using the Pemberton Happiness Index scores

reported a higher degree of well-being than Asians in retrospective global reports of well-being (i.e., remembered well-being), but there were no cultural differences in current well-being assessed by a daily diary or using an online measure.

In sum, these initial results support the existence of differences between Western and Eastern countries regarding how well-being is measured, and further it constitutes additional evidence of the PHI's construct validity.

Conclusions

It is already clear to researchers in the field of culture and well-being that it is necessary to move beyond understanding the demographics of happiness and its association with other variables (e.g., wealth and education) toward analyzing the specific mechanisms and causal influences of well-being. But it is also true that we still need good measures of well-being that can capture essential aspects of what constitutes a good life.

As we have demonstrated in this chapter, subtle methodological issues (e.g., retrospective vs. experienced well-being) may open new ways to identify critical cultural differences. As Oishi (2010) stated, "discrepancies between specific/online subjective reports and global reports of well-being seem to reflect the fact that subjective well-being is not a unitary construct" (p. 53). Well-being is a complex concept, and it would be naïve to think that single questions, notwithstanding their importance in the development of the field so far, can thoroughly grasp human happiness. The measurement of well-being includes or should include not only multiple areas of assessment but also different time frames of measurement.

In this chapter, we have presented some initial data on the PHI, a new, short index with promising psychometric data that has been initially validated using data from different countries and languages. We are aware that this is only a modest contribution to the field, but we tackled both its construction and validation while keeping in mind some of the current methodological limitations of existing measures.

More importantly, our measure was intended to overcome each of the challenges raised in the first part of this chapter. First, the PHI was designed taking into account prevailing controversies on the eudaemonic versus hedonic distinction and other current, major proposals of well-being and positive mental health. In consequence, this instrument covers the main domains of well-being described in current theories and research in the area. Moreover, as the PHI is multifaceted, it overcomes the problem of relying on concepts that are not culturally consistent such as well-being or happiness. Second, it integrates the remembered versus experienced approach to overcome the problem of how the method affects well-being scores in Western versus Eastern countries. Third, the measure itself is relatively brief considering the wide range of content that it contains.

Beyond these aspects, the PHI also presents methodological features that deserve attention. For example, all items included in the scale were empirically selected after analyzing their correlations with widely used measures of each well-being domain. Furthermore, the study sample was also larger and more multicultural than previous validation studies of similar brief scales. It is too soon to know whether this new measure will be useful in detecting and exploring significant cultural differences in well-being. Yet overall, the initial data are very encouraging (Hervas and Vazquez 2012).

Relations between cultural and individual traits, behaviors, and emotions are particularly complex (see an excellent review in Benet-Martinez and Oishi 2008). The PHI is a measure that reflects a certain point of view on well-being, which is of course, one among many possibilities. As Helliwell and Barrington-Leigh (2010) have stated, each measure reflects the preferences of its proponents. It could be possible, for instance, to design measures with different components (e.g., measures of states of calm, relaxation, peace, pride, or guilt), which research on cross-cultural differences has shown weigh differently on personal happiness or life satisfaction in different cultures (Scollon et al. 2011; Tsai et al. 2006).[8] Likewise, the concept and dimensions of social well-being (Keyes and Annas 2009) are richer than what is

---

[8] Pride and guilt are good examples of emotions that are relevant yet included neither in the PHI nor in many well-being scales. Using ESM, Scollon et al. (2004) found that Asian Americans, Indians in India, and Japanese in Japan all reported less pride and more guilt than European Americans and Hispanic Americans. Furthermore, whereas the authors did not find cross-cultural variability in sadness, the cross-cultural variability was three times greater for guilt and more than 10 times greater for pride.

addressed by our scale. Thus, the PHI is perhaps a significant contribution to the field but is in no way a definite measurement of well-being.

A final coda comments on the use of measures of well-being to establish rankings of nations. First of all, no measure can be constructed from a value-free platform. Researchers depart from different cultural traditions, and the selection of items and the weight given to them can be critical in determining the scope and sensitivity of the instrument. Furthermore, there are many alternative indices of well-being that pay attention to political or social issues that are sometimes neglected in current research in the field (e.g., ecological footprint) and may have a global impact on the current and future well-being of humans (Abdallah et al. 2008). We hope that this chapter can somehow contribute to this debate and that, above all, it has helped the reader to be more sensitive to crucial issues that are still open on the measurement of integrative well-being.

References

Abdallah, S., Thompson, S., & Marks, N. (2008). Estimating worldwide life satisfaction. *Ecological Economics, 65*, 35–47.

Benet-Martinez, V., & Oishi, S. (2008). Culture and personality. In O. P. John, R. W. Robins, & L. A. Pervin (Eds.), *Handbook of personality: Theory and research* (pp. 542–567). New York: Guilford.

Cantril, H. (1965). *The pattern of human concern*. New Brunswick: Rutgers University Press.

Cummins, R. A. (2006). *Personal Wellbeing Index – Adult* (4th ed.). The International Wellbeing Group. Melbourne: Australian Centre on Quality of Life, Deakin University.

Cummins, R. A., & Nistico, H. (2002). Maintaining life satisfaction: The role of positive cognitive bias. *Journal of Happiness Studies, 3*, 37–69.

Deaton, A. (2008). Income, health, and well-being around the world: Evidence from the Gallup World Poll. *Journal of Economic Perspectives, 22*, 53–72.

Deaton, A. (2011). *The financial crisis and the well-being of Americans*. National Bureau of Economic Research (Working Paper 17128). Retrieved October 10, 2011 from http://www.nber.org/papers/w17128

Delle Fave, A., & Bassi, M. (2009). The contribution of diversity to happiness research. *The Journal of Positive Psychology, 4*, 205–207.

Diaz, H., Horcajo, J., & Blanco, A. (2009). Development of an implicit overall well-being measure using the Implicit Association Test. *Spanish Journal of Psychology, 12*, 604–617.

Diener, E. (1984). Subjective well-being. *Psychological Bulletin, 95*, 542–575.

Diener, E. (2000). Subjective well-being: The science of happiness, and a proposal for a national index. *American Psychologist, 55*, 34–43.

Diener, E., & Chan, M. (2011). Happy people live longer: Subjective well-being contributes to health and longevity. *Applied Psychology: Health and Well-Being, 3*, 1–43.

Diener, E., & Suh, E. M. (2000). *Culture and subjective well-being*. Cambridge: The MIT Press.

Diener, E., & Seligman, M. E. P. (2002). Very happy people. *Psychological Science, 13*, 81–84.

Diener, E., Emmons, R. A., Larsen, R. J., & Griffin, S. (1985). The satisfaction with life scale. *Journal of Personality Assessment, 49*, 71–75.

Diener, E., Scollon, C. K., Oishi, S., Dzokoto, V., & Suh, E. M. (2000). Positivity and the construction of life satisfaction judgments: Global happiness is not the sum of its parts. *Journal of Happiness Studies, 1*, 159–176.

Diener, E., Oishi, S., & Lucas, R. E. (2003). Personality, culture, and subjective well-being: Emotional and cognitive evaluations of life. *Annual Review of Psychology, 54*, 403–425.

Diener, E., Wirtz, D., Tov, W., Kim-Prieto, C., Choi, D., Oishi, S., & Biswas-Diener, R. (2009). New well-being measures: Short scales to assess flourishing and positive and negative feelings. *Social Indicators Research, 97*, 143–156.

Diener, E., Kahneman, D., Tov, W., & Arora, R. (2010). Income's association with judgments of life versus feelings. In E. Diener, J. Helliwell, & D. Kahneman (Eds.), *International differences in well-being* (pp. 3–15). New York: Oxford University Press.

Eid, M. (2008). Measuring the immeasurable: Psychometric modeling of subjective well-being data. In M. Eid & R. Larsen (Eds.), *The science of subjective well-being* (pp. 141–169). New York: Guilford.

Eid, M., & Diener, E. (2001). Norms for experiencing emotions in different cultures: Inter-and intranational differences. *Journal of Personality and Social Psychology, 81*, 869–885.

Harter, J. K., & Gurley, V. (2008). Measuring well-being in the United States. *Association for Psychological Science Observer, 21*(8). Retrieved from http://www.psychologicalscience.org/observer/getArticle.cfm?id=2394

Helliwell, J. F., & Barrington-Leigh, C. P. (2010). Measuring and understanding subjective well-being. *Canadian Journal of Economics, 43*, 729–753.

Hervas, G., & Vazquez, C. (2010). *Remembering and experiencing well-being: Results from an international study.* Paper presented at the 5th European Conference on Positive Psychology, Copenhagen, June 2010.

Hervas, C., & Vazquez, C. (2012). *Validation of a brief measure of integrative well-being in seven languages: The Pemberton Happiness Index.* Submitted for publication.

Huebner, E. S., Gilman, R., & Laughlin, J. (1999). The multidimensionality of children's well-being reports: Discriminant validity of life satisfaction and self-esteem. *Social Indicators Research, 46*, 1–22.

Kahneman, D. (1999). Objective happiness. In E. Diener, N. Schwarz, & D. Kahneman (Eds.), *Well-being: The foundations of hedonic psychology* (pp. 3–25). New York: Russell Sage.

Kahneman, D., & Krueger, A. B. (2006). Developments in the measurement of subjective well-being. *Journal of Economic Perspectives, 20*, 3–24.

Kahneman, D., Krueger, A. B., Schkade, D. A., Schwarz, N., & Stone, A. A. (2004). A survey method for characterizing daily life experience: The day reconstruction method. *Science, 306*, 1776–1780.

Kahneman, D., Krueger, A. B., Schkade, D., Schwarz, N., & Stone, A. A. (2006). Would you be happier if you were richer? A focusing illusion. *Science, 312*, 1908–1910.

Kapteyn, A., Smith, J. P., & van Soest, A. (2010). Life satisfaction. In E. Diener, J. Helliwell, & D. Kahneman (Eds.), *International differences in well-being* (pp. 70–104). New York: Oxford University Press.

Kashdan, T. B., Biswas-Diener, R., & King, L. A. (2008). Reconsidering happiness: The costs of distinguishing between hedonics and eudaimonia. *The Journal of Positive Psychology, 3*, 219–233.

Keyes, C. L. (1998). Social well-being. *Social Psychology Quarterly, 61*, 121–140.

Keyes, C. L., & Annas, J. (2009). Feeling good and functioning well: Distinctive concepts in ancient philosophy and contemporary science. *The Journal of Positive Psychology, 4*, 197–201.

Keyes, C. L., Ryff, C., & Shmotkin, D. (2002). Optimizing well-being: The empirical encounter of two traditions. *Journal of Personality and Social Psychology, 82*, 1007–1022.

Lopez, S. J., & Snyder, C. R. (Eds.). (2003). *Positive psychological assessment: A handbook of models and measures.* Washington, DC: American Psychological Association.

Lu, L., & Gilmour, R. (2004). Culture and conceptions of happiness: Individual oriented and social oriented subjective well-being. *Journal of Happiness Studies, 5*, 269–291.

Lucas, R. E., Diener, E., & Suh, E. (1996). Discriminant validity of well-being measures. *Journal of Personality and Social Psychology, 71*, 616–628.

Lyubomirsky, S., & Lepper, H. S. (1999). A measure of subjective happiness: Preliminary reliability and construct validation. *Social Indicators Research, 46*, 137–155.

Lyubomirsky, S., King, L., & Diener, E. (2005). The benefits of frequent positive affect: Does happiness lead to success? *Psychological Bulletin, 131*, 803–855.

Mesquita, B., & Leu, J. (2007). The cultural psychology of emotion. In S. Kitayama & D. Cohen (Eds.), *Handbook of cultural psychology* (pp. 734–759). New York: Guilford.

Morrison, M., Tay, L., & Diener, E. (2011). Subjective well-being and national satisfaction: Findings from a worldwide survey. *Psychological Science, 22*, 166–171.

Oishi, S. (2002). The experiencing and remembering of well-being: A cross cultural analysis. *Personality and Social Psychology Bulletin, 28*, 1398–1406.

Oishi, S. (2010). Culture and well-being: Conceptual and methodological issues. In E. Diener, D. Kahneman, & J. F. Helliwell, (Eds.), *International differences in well-being* (pp. 34–69). New York: Oxford University Press.

Oishi, S., & Diener, E. (2003). Culture and well-being: The cycle of action, evaluation and decision. *Personality and Social Psychology Bulletin, 28*, 1398–1406.

Oishi, S., & Schimmack, U. (2010). Culture and well-being: A new inquiry into the psychological wealth of nations. *Perspectives on Psychological Science, 5*, 463–471.

Oswald, A. J., & Wu, S. (2010). Objective confirmation of subjective measures of human well-being: Evidence from the USA. *Science, 327*, 576–579.

Reis, H. T., & Gable, S. L. (2000). Event-sampling and other methods for studying everyday experience. In H. T. Reis & C. M. Judd (Eds.), *Handbook of research methods in social and personality psychology* (pp. 190–222). New York: Cambridge University Press.

Russell, J. A. (1991). Culture and the categorization of emotion. *Psychological Bulletin, 110*, 426–450.

Ryan, R. M., & Deci, E. L. (2001). On happiness and human potential: A review of research on hedonic and eudaimonic well-being. *Annual Review of Psychology, 52*, 141–166.

Ryan, R. M., & Frederick, C. M. (1997). On energy, personality, and health: Subjective vitality as a dynamic reflection of well-being. *Journal of Personality, 65*, 529–565.

Ryan, R. M., & Huta, V. (2009). Wellness as healthy functioning or wellness as happiness: The importance of eudaimonic thinking. *The Journal of Positive Psychology, 4*, 202–204.

Ryff, C. D. (1989). Happiness is everything, or is it? Explorations on the meaning of psychological well-being. *Journal of Personality and Social Psychology, 57*, 1069–1081.

Ryff, C. D., & Keyes, C. L. (1995). The structure of psychological well-being revisited. *Journal of Personality and Social Psychology, 69*, 719–727.

Schimmack, U., Radhakrishnan, P., Oishi, S., Dzokoto, V., & Ahadi, S. (2002). Culture, personality, and subjective well-being: Integrating process models of life satisfaction. *Journal of Personality and Social Psychology, 82*, 582–593.

Schimmack, U., Oishi, S., & Diener, E. (2005). Individualism: A valid and important dimension of cultural differences between nations. *Personality and Social Psychology Review, 9*, 17–31.

Schwarz, N. (1999). Self-reports: How the questions shape the answers. *American Psychologist, 54*, 93–105.

Scollon, C. N., Kim-Prieto, C., & Diener, E. (2003). Experience sampling: Promises and pitfalls, strengths and weaknesses. *Journal of Happiness Studies, 4*, 5–34.

Scollon, C. N., Diener, E., Oishi, S., & Biswas-Diener, R. (2004). Emotions across cultures and methods. *Journal of Cross-Cultural Psychology, 35*, 304–326.

Scollon, C. N., Howard, A. H., Caldwell, A. E., & Ito, S. (2009). The role of ideal affect in the experience and memory of emotions. *Journal of Happiness Studies, 10*, 257–269.

Scollon, C. N., Koh, S., & Au, E. (2011). Cultural differences in the subjective experience of emotion: When and why they occur. *Personality and Social Psychology Compass, 5*, 853–864.

Stewart-Brown, S., Tennant, A., Tennant, R., Platt, S., Parkinson, J., & Weich, S. (2009). Internal construct validity of the Warwick-Edinburgh Mental Well-being Scale (WEMWBS): A Rasch analysis using data from the Scottish Health Education Population Survey. *Health and Quality of Life Outcomes, 7*, 15. doi:10.1186/1477-7525-7-15.

Suh, E. M., & Koo, J. (2008). Comparing subjective well-being across cultures and nations: The "what" and "why" questions. In M. Eid & R. J. Larsen (Eds.), *The science of subjective well-being* (pp. 414–427). New York: Guilford Press.

Tamir, M., & Gross, J. J. (2011). Beyond pleasure and pain? Emotion regulation and positive psychology. In K. Sheldon, T. Kashdan, & M. Steger (Eds.), *Designing the future of positive psychology: Taking stock and moving forward* (pp. 89–100). New York: Oxford University Press.

Tennant, R., Hiller, L., Fishwick, R., Platt, S., Joseph, S., Weich, S., Parkinson, J., Secker, S., & Stewart-Brown, S. (2007). The Warwick-Edinburgh Mental Well-Being Scale (WEMWBS): Development and UK validation. *Health and Quality of Life Outcomes, 5*, 63. doi:10.1186/1477-7525-5-63.

Tov, W., & Diener, E. (2007). Culture and subjective well-being. In S. Kitayama & D. Cohen (Eds.), *Handbook of cultural psychology* (pp. 691–713). New York: Guilford.

Tsai, J. L., Knutson, B., & Fung, H. H. (2006). Cultural variation in affect valuation. *Journal of Personality and Social Psychology, 90*, 288–307.

van Hemert, D. A., Poortinga, Y. H., & van de Vijver, F. J. R. (2007). Emotion and culture. A meta-analysis. *Cognition and Emotion, 21*, 913–943.

Vargas, H. (2010). *Estudio de los conceptos cotidianos de happiness y felicidad desde un enfoque probabilístico* (Doctoral dissertation). Universidad Autonoma de Madrid. [*A study on the concepts of 'happiness' and 'felicidad' from a probabilistic framework*]. Retrieved June 1, 2012 from http://www.tesisenred.net/handle/10803/50782

Vázquez, C., Hervás, G., Rahona, J. J., & Gómez, D. (2009). Psychological well-being and health: Contributions of positive psychology. *Annuary of Clinical and Health Psychology, 5*, 15–28.

Vázquez, C., Rahona, J. J., Gómez, D., & Hervás, G., (2011). *Mind over matter: A national representative study of the relative impact of physical and psychological problems on life satisfaction*. Submitted for publication.

Veenhoven, R. (2000). Wellbeing in the welfare state: Level not higher, distribution not more equitable. *Journal of Comparative Policy Analysis, 2*, 91–125.

Veenhoven, R. (2007). Measures of gross national happiness. In OECD: Statistics, knowledge and policy. Measuring and fostering the progress of societies (2007), pp. 231–253. Retrieved on June 15th, 2012 from: http://mpra.ub.uni-muenchen.de/11280/

Veenhoven, R. (2009). How universal is happiness? In E. Diener, J. Helliwell, & D. Kahneman (Eds.), *International differences in well-being* (pp. 328–350). New York: Oxford University Press.

Veenhoven, R. (2011). *World database of happiness, ongoing register of scientific research on subjective enjoyment of life*. http://worlddatabaseofhappiness.eur.nl

Vitterso, J., Biswas-Diener, R., & Diener, E. (2005). The divergent meaning of life satisfaction: Item response modeling of the satisfaction with life scale in Greenland and Norway. *Social Indicators Research, 74*, 327–348.

Waterman, A. S. (2008). Reconsidering happiness: A eudaimonist's perspective. *The Journal of Positive Psychology, 3*, 234–252.

Watson, D., Clark, L. A., & Tellegen, A. (1988). Development and validation of brief measures of positive and negative affect: The PANAS scales. *Journal of Personality and Social Psychology, 54*, 1063–1070.

Wirtz, D., Kruger, J., Scollon, C. N., & Diener, E. (2003). What to do on spring break? Predicting future choice based on online versus recalled affect. *Psychological Science, 14*, 520–524.

Xu, J., & Roberts, R. E. (2010). The power of positive emotions: it's a matter of life or death: Subjective well-being and longevity over 28 years in a general population. *Health Psychology, 29*, 9–19.

Yamaguchi, S., Greenwald, A. G., Banaji, M. R., Murakami, F., Chen, D., Shiomura, K., et al. (2007). Apparent universality of positive implicit self-esteem. *Psychological Science, 18*, 498–500.

Chapter 4
Communal Values and Individualism in Our Era of Globalization: A Comparative Longitudinal Study of Three Different Societies

Hilde Eileen Nafstad, Rolv Mikkel Blakar, Albert Botchway, Erlend Sand Bruer, Petra Filkukova, and Kim Rand-Hendriksen

Introduction[1]

As human beings, we cannot provide the context for our well-being entirely by ourselves. Each of us is dependent on other people's care and civic virtues. Thus, the well-being and good life of the individual is deeply tied to the well-being of others and positive social institutions. Participation in shared or common goods grows out of our social nature: our dispositions for empathy and civility (Batson 1991; Hoffman 1975; Peterson and Seligman 2004). At the same time, the cultural level with its ethics ideologies shapes our social and empathic dispositions as we take part in practices and custom complexes of our culture.

Therefore, in every culture, there has to be a powerful set of ideals about collectivism and individualism; societies have to find a balance between individual independence and collective interdependence. Thus, conceptions of what makes a good life have, in essential and fundamental ways, to consider both individual autonomy and personal growth and the individual's partaking in developing, upholding,

---

[1] As the present study is conducted as an integrated part of a comparative research program, it is inevitable that the theoretical-methodological framework has been presented in former articles and reports from the project.

H.E. Nafstad (✉)
Department of Psychology and Centre for the Study of Mind in Nature (CSMN),
University of Oslo, PO Box 1094, Blindern, 0317 Oslo, Norway
e-mail: h.e.nafstad@psykologi.uio.no

R.M. Blakar • E.S. Bruer • P. Filkukova
Department of Psychology, University of Oslo, Oslo, Norway

A. Botchway
Department of Psychology, Southern Illinois University at Carbondale, Oslo, Norway

K. Rand-Hendriksen
Department of Health Management and Health Economics Medical Faculty,
University of Oslo, Oslo, Norway

H.H. Knoop and A. Delle Fave (eds.), *Well-Being and Cultures: Perspectives from Positive Psychology*, Cross-Cultural Advancements in Positive Psychology 3, DOI 10.1007/978-94-007-4611-4_4, © Springer Science+Business Media Dordrecht 2013

and maintaining his or her community (Nafstad et al. 2009a). Based on its own local historical and cultural traditions, every society has, therefore, to negotiate its own balance between individual and communal values. During the last decades, the degree of interconnections between various world regions has, due to modern communications and economic and financial interdependence between continents and regions, strongly accelerated. Conceiving globalization as an ideology or world-view, as a system of ideas and values circulating in the public realm influencing societies worldwide thereby defining and articulating local values and visions for social change, this study analyzes the influences of globalization on individualism, communal values, and sense of community in three different societies: a post-communist Eastern European state (the Czech Republic), a Nordic welfare state (Norway) and a modern West African society (Ghana).

Currently, late capitalist market ideology is spreading across the globe. This ideology or worldview is based strongly on excessive individualism (Bauman 2000; Giddens 1991; Nafstad et al. 2007, 2009b; Stiglitz 2002). Thereby, there is a danger of neglecting the human being as a social and civic virtuous person capable of empathy and concern for others and the common good (Batson 1991; Hoffman 2000; Nafstad 2005). Thus, across the world, current meaning structures of good life and well-being may be increasingly dominated by a strong, monolithic ideal or value of self-fulfillment: almost the ideal of egotism. We are supposed to expose our selfish concerns. Are today's public discourses around the world, therefore, moving away from the ideal of commitments to others and toward self-centeredness, entitlements, and asocial egoism? Are public discourses around the world currently moving away from an ideal of a careful balance between individual interests and moral visions of fundamental social responsibility and acceptance of others and community? These are the questions raised in this chapter.

The Concept of Ideology and the Ideology of Neoliberalism

Ideologies are associated with socially shared ideas or beliefs (Billig 1997; Nafstad et al. 2012; Van Dijk 1998). Ideology is thus a *Weltanschauung* constituted by cultural values that are taken for granted and shared by members of a society or group. Consequently, ideologies function as cultural structures of meaning, ideals, and norms in society and provide organizing principles for actions of individuals, groups, and institutions (Nafstad et al. 2006, 2009c). An ideology is thus an important meaning system that describes for the individual both the world that *is* and prescribes the world that *ought to be* (Wilson 1992).

As Sampson (1981: 731) contends, on the intra-psychological level, the concept of ideology refers to "… the ideas and thoughts that people hold, including both the form and content of their consciousness." At the same time, ideologies are, as emphasized, socially constructed collective representations or collective voices, as their origin is cultural and they are shared by a large number of individuals. Furthermore, ideologies are discursively mediated in that they are typically expressed in everyday media and professional language (Bakhtin 1952/1986; Blakar 1973/2006, 1979; Mutz 1998).

Media language is presently of particular importance due to the increasing role of mass media as the major "machineries of meaning" (Hermans and Kempen 1998). By being exposed to such languages, the individual becomes attuned to and incorporates the currently predominant ideologies of society. Operating in a globalized context, contemporary media strongly contribute toward creating and shaping our ideologies, both as producers and mediators of these ideologies. Consequently, it is increasingly likely to find all over the world a widespread awareness of a larger world culture (Skrbis et al. 2004). Globalized ideologies mediated by mass media thus increasingly integrate and interconnect societies and organizations all over the world.

Currently, the late capitalist market ideology is spreading across the globe (Arnett 2002; Chryssochoou 2004). This ideology is, as mentioned, based on free-market principles and excessive individualism, strongly promoting each individual's freedom to choose and to make his/her choices in a manner aiming to maximize acquisition of material and nonmaterial goods, primarily for oneself. Thus, this globalized ideology emphasizes the values of radical or excessive individualism. In so doing, there is a danger of neglecting communal values and the conception of the human being as a civic virtuous person with a psychological sense of solidarity and community (Batson 1991; Hoffman 1975, 2000; Nafstad 2002, 2005). Thus, current meaning structures of personal identity, good life, and happiness around the world may be predominated by a strong ideal or value of self-fulfillment: Humans are supposed to expose their selfish concerns. Therefore, our sense of prosociality and our willingness to take responsibility for other persons, to act for the common good, and to accept and defend collective rights and interests may be increasingly difficult to nurture in contemporary societies all over the world. We contend that the current neoliberalist variant of capitalism, with its excessive individualist ideology, is becoming increasingly more influential, profoundly affecting local worldviews of good life and well-being.

Ideologies and Language Usage

Linguists, social scientists, and psychologists have for a long time acknowledged the close and reciprocal relations between language and ideology (cf., Nafstad et al. 2012). Primarily, it has been linguistically oriented anthropologists that have endeavored to investigate this interplay between language and ideology (cf., Kroskrity 2000). Silverstein (1985) emphasized the reciprocal interaction between language and ideology: "... the total linguistic fact, the datum for a science of language, is irreducibly dialectic in nature. It is an unstable mutual interaction of meaningful sign forms contextualized to situations of interested human use and mediated by the fact of cultural ideology" (p. 220). It is this contextualization and mediation through cultural ideology which renders language, indeed even the single word (Blakar 1973/2006, 1979; Pennebaker et al. 2003; Rommetveit 1968; Rommetveit and Blakar 1979), into very precise and undisguised reflections of a given society and enables analysis of ideological influence on the individual. Changes in language use over time may therefore reflect profound macrosocial or ideological developments (Blakar 1973/2006, 1979).

In order to describe ideologies, then, words and expressions constitute useful analytical units (Nafstad et al. 2007, 2009b, c). They can represent empirical indicators of the ideological situation, of adjustments and pressures. Negotiations and recalibrations serving to maintain or to construe new value systems and interpretative repertoires can thus be revealed in linguistic changes over time. Analyses of key words, expressions, and utterances thus constitute a valid method to describe how ideological discourses in different cultures develop and change, for instance, under the pressure of currently globalized neoliberalism.

Individualism and Communal Values in an Era of Globalization

Collectivism and individualism are perhaps the most frequently examined cultural characteristics (Hofstede 1991; Triandis 1990, 1995; Triandis and Trafimov 2001). The collectivist ideology emphasizes groups, other people, and community, while individualism is based on concerns for oneself and one's immediate family. Both of the ideologies or worldviews, we contend, are essential in society. They are life-oriented ideals for individual and community and therefore important to know about for positive psychology. However, mixtures of collectivism and individualism will develop as societies continually create amalgamations of individual and collective goals and thereby standards for the optimal functioning a person is expected to achieve (Ryan et al. 1999). In a former study (Nafstad et al. 2009a), it was demonstrated how West African Ghana and North European Norway responded systematically different to the strong individualism imbued in currently globalizing ideologies. As expected, in both societies, individualist values were markedly strengthened under the influence of globalization during the past decades. However, whereas communal ideals or values decreased markedly in Norway, communal values increased in Ghana. We will now follow up this study with analyses of a society very different from both Ghana and Norway. We will analyze ideological and value developments across time in the Czech Republic and compare with developmental trends of collectivism and individualism in Ghana, a modern West African society, and Norway, a Nordic welfare state. The Czech Republic is of particular interest as the former Czechoslovakia was part of the communist Eastern Europe and has undergone profound changes after the Iron Curtain was lifted. Therefore, the Czech Republic has been in a situation of transformation where ideals for individual and cultural practices most probably have to be reformulated.

The Czech Republic, Ghana, and Norway

A North European, post-industrial, and (historically) protestant nation with good and stable economic conditions, Norway, as one of the Scandinavian welfare states, has traditionally been characterized by an ideology valuing social equality, social obligation, and universalistic principles for distribution of common goods. Thus, there has traditionally been a strong emphasis to value collective arrangements and equal distribution of public services and common goods (Carlquist et al. 2007). We have, in previous studies, analyzed ideological changes which have taken place in the Norwegian society over the past 25 years, from 1984[2] on, and have demonstrated how Norway increasingly has been imbued by the globalizing ideology of neoliberalism with its excessive individualism, in marked contrast to and exerting pressure on the collective arrangements valued by the traditional welfare state (Nafstad et al. 2006, 2007, 2009a, b, c).

A former colony of Britain, Ghana, gained its independence in 1957. Situated along the West Coast of Africa, Ghana is characterized by very challenging social and economic conditions. However, Ghana was one of the first African countries to implement economic reforms under the tutelage of the World Bank (Aryeetey et al. 2000). Akotia and Barimah (2007) contend that traditional Ghanaian values in general "... prescribe collectivism and social support for each other. ... Every individual in the community has the social responsibility for the other person" (p. 410). This collectivistic worldview is captured in the statement: "I am because we are, and because we are, therefore I am" (Akotia and Olowu 2000, p. 4). This attitude may explain why we found communal values to be increasing in Ghana (Nafstad et al. 2009a).

Czechoslovakia was created in 1918, following the collapse of the Austro-Hungarian Empire. In 1948, the Communist Party took control, and the country became part of the Eastern Bloc. In 1989, Czechoslovakia changed from a communist regime to liberal democracy, during the so-called Velvet Revolution. The Czech Republic was created in 1993 when Czechoslovakia peacefully split into two independent states: the Czech Republic and Slovakia (Agnew 2008). Thus, Czech ideology has been deeply marked by 41 years of communist rule, leading to a situation where individuals are unwilling to take responsibility for decisions, political or other (Švejnar and Hvížďala 2008). Social responsibility was, during communist rule, conceived of as an entirely collective matter. There is currently a growing public dissatisfaction with the inability of Czech politicians to deal with what is perceived as a system of "wild capitalism" and widespread corruption. The societal ideologies in the Czech Republic has thus undergone profound changes over the past decades, from communist regime to modern democracy and to "wild capitalism." The country is now continually struggling to deal with these huge transitions of ideologies and value systems concerning collective and individualist rights, entitlements, and duties.

Given the currently globalizing neoliberalism, we expect that individualist values will be increasing in the Czech Republic as well as in the other two societies. However, given the dramatic changes the Czech Republic has undergone during the past years after the fall of the Iron Curtain, we expect a mixed pattern of collective and individualist values and less clear-cut developmental trends, in particular with regard to communal values, compared to Norway and Ghana. Even though we are now analyzing a slightly different period of time, there is

---

[2] Newspapers in Norway have been electronically filed and thereby accessible for analysis since 1984.

every reason to assume that the developmental patterns in Ghana and Norway with regard to individualism and communal values will still be as described above (cf. Nafstad et al. 2009a).

Method

A Longitudinal Design

The present study is based on a longitudinal design, identifying ideology and ideological shifts as reflected in electronically archived media (newspaper) language from the time when searchable electronic archives were established to present. For the Norwegian society, we have during the past decade developed and refined a methodology for assessing and describing developmental trends over time (from 1984 when the first Norwegian newspaper became electronically available, see method section).[3] The searching facilities and methods of analyses are not as flexible in Ghana and the Czech Republic as those developed in Norway.[4] We will therefore present the methodology as used in the Norwegian analyses and point out how the methodologies available in Ghana and the Czech Republic deviate from this.

Materials: Search Words

How do we select search words? In principle, a huge variety of words and expressions of the actual language might constitute possible search words for selection (Nafstad et al. 2006, 2007, 2009a, b, c). The words used in the present study were identified by their potential contribution to the redefinition of individualist versus communal values in society. Words referring to or words denoting communality and community such as we, us, responsibility, solidarity, etc. and words indicative of individualism such as I, me, rights, etc. The principles for identifying search words in the Ghanaian and Czech analyses are, logically, the same as in the Norwegian ones. Care was taken to establish sets of words that function as equivalent as possible in the three languages: Norwegian, English (the written language in Ghana), and Czech. The Norwegian search words are presented in Table 4.1, the Ghanaian in Table 4.2, and the Czech in Table 4.3.

---

[3] The method is developed as a "mixed methodology design" (Tashakkori and Teddlie 1998) in that aspects of both the quantitative and qualitative paradigm are combined throughout most steps of the process of assessing ideological shifts. However, in large-scale mappings such as the present study, it is possible to adopt the method purely quantitatively, mapping changes in frequencies of newspaper articles using various key words over time.

[4] The methodologies used in the Ghanaian and Czech societies, however, are at about the same level of refinements as the methodology we used in the first studies in Norway.

Materials: Newspapers

An increasing number of newspapers in Norway have been digitally filed and made electronically accessible by way of a comprehensive, integrated database (Retriever) located on the World Wide Web. Thus, it is now possible to identify and trace a variety of changes in media language over time.

To ensure representativity, an array of available newspapers with differential profiles should be included when analyzing the ideological situation. Various newspapers make different ideological contributions to and reflections about society. In electronic archives, newspapers are gradually added over time. Therefore, it is easier to ensure representativity in synchronic analyses than in longitudinal or diachronic analyses to adopt Saussure's classic distinction (cf., Lyons 1968). At present, the Norwegian electronic archive covers more than 50 newspapers. Only one newspaper, the nationwide Aftenposten, has been included from the very establishment of the electronic database in 1984. As it is essential for longitudinal analyses to cover as long a time span as possible, the analysis reported here is restricted to Aftenposten, which allows analysis across more than two decades (1984–2008). Aftenposten represents a traditional broadsheet paper covering politics, national as well as international and foreign, economics, culture, and sports. Aftenposten has a somewhat conservative basic orientation. The main editorial office is located in Oslo, the capital. However, Aftenposten has local editorial offices and journalists and contributors throughout the country.[5]

As our longitudinal analyses are based on only one newspaper, *Aftenposten*, its representativity as an indicator of developmental changes in media language is critical. To assess representativity, we have conducted correlation analyses of the developmental pattern over time of the frequency of usage identified in Aftenposten for each word with the developmental pattern of frequency of usage identified in the five other newspapers available in Retriever since 1992,[6] combined. Only search words for which the developmental trend in *Aftenposten* correlates significantly (at .05 level) with that of the other five newspapers combined for the period 1992 through 2008, i.e., more than two-thirds of the total period analyzed, should be included. Neither in Ghana nor in the Czech Republic existed integrated databases allowing such refined procedures for assessing reliability of the chosen newspaper.

There are two potential sources of error one must control for when mapping changes over time. First, there is variation in the total number of articles published within newspapers from year to year. Second, the average length of a newspaper

---

[5] During our research period, Retriever expanded the database; the tabloid VG was by scanning made available as far back as 1945. However, due to both theoretical issues and methodological instabilities, we have not included VG further back than 1992 as one of five newspapers used for assessing Aftenposten's reliability (see below).

[6] The five newspapers are *Bergens Tidende, Dagens Næringsliv, Nordlys, NTB*, and *VG*. These newspapers hold different editorial positions on political and ideological issues, and NTB is a press agency delivering articles to all Norwegian newspapers.

article may also vary by year. Thus, as newspapers publish a different number of total articles that vary in length in any given year, a baseline adjustment has to be administered in order to examine and compare developmental trends over time. As an empirical adjustment factor, we use the average development of the 10,000 most frequently used words in the Norwegian language (Rand-Hendriksen 2008). Neither in Ghana nor in the Czech Republic was it possible to adopt such a refined procedure. In both countries, mean number of articles published annually in the actual newspaper during the period analyzed is used as basis for adjusting scores.

Percentages of changes in the usage of words from 1984 to 2008 give an understandable expression of the magnitude of changes. However, there are limitations in using mere percentages for analytical purposes: First, for new words and expressions being introduced during the period, it is impossible to calculate percentage increase (as the baseline is zero). Second, for words and expressions with infrequent usage, the percentage change may be several hundred and thus not representative. Third, the percentage rate of change does not differentiate between a gradual change over the whole period of time, or, for example, an abrupt increase the very last year. Fourth, percentage change increase and decrease of usage function differently: A decrease cannot exceed 100%, whereas there is in principle no limit to how many percent the usage of a word or utterance may increase. Fifth, and most importantly, it is difficult to compare magnitudes of change detected in newspapers that have been electronically available for different periods of time. To meet these obstacles, we adopted the following unit to express trend change over time: "estimated mean annual change" (EMAC). To calculate EMAC, we start with the slope of the linear regression line. To turn the slope into a measure comparable for different time spans and different absolute levels, we calculate a relative slope. To obtain the relative slope, rather than the absolute gradient of the regression line, one would normally base the calculation on the score of the first observation (the first year of the time series). As the score for the first year in our analysis may be zero (i.e., for new words that are introduced during the period), we have based our calculations on the average number of articles per year during the entire period covered in investigation. In addition to always being above zero, the average is more resistant to random fluctuation than any single measure. To obtain EMAC, we therefore divide the slope (change per year according to linear regression) by average score (average number of articles per year) and then multiply by 100, which yields the mean annual percentage change.

A developmental trend can also be described in terms of how strongly the developmental pattern for a particular word (the time series data) correlates with the annual time series itself (1984, 1985, ..., 2008); this will give correlation with linear time.

In Ghana and the Czech Republic, there exists no integrated, searchable database similar to the Norwegian Retriever. However, in Ghana, a searchable electronic news archive containing selected articles from various Ghanaian newspapers is available in the form of GhanaWeb. This news archive is thus an edited archive and does not cover complete newspaper output. Still, this archive includes articles from the main Ghanaian newspapers and covers a broad range of issues: from politics and economics to culture, religion, and sports. GhanaWeb goes back to 1995. However, in 1995 and particularly in 1996, few articles are included. Consequently, it was decided to use 1997 as the starting year in order to obtain reliable results. A growing number of newspapers are being made available electronically in the Czech Republic. The second largest newspaper,[7] *Mladá fronta DNES*, was chosen because it was the first Czech newspaper available in a searchable electronic database. Historically, this paper used to be the mouthpiece of the Czech Communist Party's Socialist Youth, but its journalists were among the first to challenge censorship and cover the Czech Velvet Revolution. After the revolution, the word "dnes" (Czech for "today") was added to the title of the newspaper, signifying end of state ownership and censorship of the newspaper. The archive goes back to 1996, but due to great fluctuations in total number of articles in the first years (1996–1998), we decided to use 1999 as the starting year.

In the Norwegian database Retriever, Boolean functions such as OR, AND, AND NOT, and so on can be used to identify articles containing, for example, either of the words x OR y. Articles containing either "jeg" (I) OR "meg" (me) or articles containing both "likhet" (equality) AND "rettferdighet" (justice) can thus be identified. Moreover, in the Norwegian database, there exists a truncation function, enabling identification of every word/utterance starting with a specified string of letters. This means that a search word in Norwegian is being identified in all forms (singular and plural, definite and indefinite, as part of a longer compound word, and so on) in one single truncated search. In GhanaWeb, neither Boolean functions nor truncation is available. Only single words or utterances (word strings) can be searched in GhanaWeb. The search functions of Mladá fronta DNES allows the Boolean function OR and truncation. However, due to the complexity of the Czech grammar, adopting truncation would have resulted in a lot of search results not comparable to the Norwegian and Ghanaian search words. It should also be mentioned that the language situation in Ghana is complex; a series of local languages are spoken, whereas English is the official language. English is also the language of GhanaWeb.

The developmental patterns found in Aftenposten correlate significantly with the developmental pattern identified in the five other newspapers combined at the .05 level for all but three of the words and at .01 level for two-thirds of the words.[8] We are confident, therefore, that the patterns of change in language usage that we identify are representative of Norwegian media language, at least from 1992 to 2008. There should

---

[7] The second largest newspaper was chosen instead of the largest Czech newspaper, "Blesk," because Blesk was regarded as too tabloid compared to the archives chosen in Norway and Ghana. Comparison between archives could have been difficult if the selected newspapers varied too greatly in journalistic style.

[8] The three search words included, even though the developmental patterns in Aftenposten do not correlate significantly with the other newspapers, are: *ansvar* (responsibility), *rettferdighet* (justice), and *borgere* (citizens). They are included because they represent very interesting issues in comparative analyses. When discussing trends in the Norwegian society, these three search words have to be interpreted with greater care than the others.

be no reason to assume a different situation in the pre-1992 period. Whereas we are confident about the representativity of our analyses of changes in language usage in Norwegian newspapers, we are thus less certain about the representativity of our analyses of changes in Ghanaian and Czech public discourses.

Results: Presentation and Discussion

To best capture potential influences of globalization processes over the past decades, we start by presenting data from Norway where a period of 25 years is covered. We then present developmental trends in Ghana and the Czech Republic where much shorter periods are covered. Finally, developmental trends for all three countries for the decade 1999–2008, the time period covered in all three countries, are compared.

Norway (1984–2008)

Developmental changes over time for the various words in the Norwegian context are presented in Table 4.1. The marked increase (55%) of articles, including either "*jeg*" OR "*meg*" (I OR me) compared to the more stable pattern (16% increase) for articles containing either "*vi*" OR "*oss*" (we OR us), is a strong indication of a shift toward increased individualism. Another indication of shifts toward more individualist values in the Norwegian society is demonstrated by a 38% increase of articles including the word "*rettighet*" (rights; entitlements), whereas there is a 35% decrease of articles containing the word "*plikt*" (duty; obligation). The developmental trends of the usage of both these words correlate significantly with linear time (see Table 4.1). Add to these findings that the usage of the word "*solidaritet*" (solidarity) during the same period has been reduced by 61%. Furthermore, the above descriptions of the ideological shifts are underlined in that individuals are conceptualized increasingly as "*brukere*" (users; consumers); the usage of the word "*brukere*" has increased 77%, and the developmental trend correlates significantly with linear time. At the same time, there have been only minor changes in the usage of the word "*borgere*" (citizens) (see Table 4.1).

Our analysis also reveals an unequivocal decline in the usage of a number of words and concepts which may be connected to communality. The usage of the word "*felles*" (common; communality; shared) has decreased by 27%. The reduction in frequency of usage correlates significantly with linear time with an estimated mean annual change (EMAC) of −2.0% during the 25-year period. Moreover, the usage of the words "*samhold*" and "*samhørighet*," both referring to social cohesion and belongingness, declined by 34% and 65%, respectively. For these two words, the reduction in frequency of usage correlates significantly with linear time with EMACs of respectively −3.2% and −5.1%.

Table 4.1 The search words used in the longitudinal (1984–2008) analysis in the Norwegian society with number of articles observed in 2008[a], percentage increase/decrease since 1984, correlations (Pearson's r) with linear time (year), and estimated mean annual change (EMAC) for each search word. Data for the comparative 1999–2008 period is included as well

Search word	Adjusted no. occurrences in 2008	Percent increase/decrease since 1984/1999		Correlation with linear time (year) 1984–2008/1999–2008		Estimated mean annual change (EMAC) (in %) 1984–2008/1999–2008	
Rettighet[b] (right; entitlement)	1,308	38	18	.88**	.81**	1.7	2.0
Plikt[b] (duty; obligation)	681	−35	−11	−0.93**	−0.51	−1.5	−1.1
Ansvar[b] (responsibility)	5,272	−13	−5	−0.87**	−0.62	−0.7	−0.9
Felles[b] (common; communal; shared)	3,722	−27	−2	−0.85**	−0.39	−1.7	−0.4
Solidaritet[b] (solidarity)	310	−61	−5	−0.90**	−0.65*	−4.5	−1.8
Samhold[b] (cohesion)	173	−34	−13	0.87**	.09	−3.2	−0.3
Samhørighet[b] (belongingness)	35	−65	−21	−0.93**	−0.20	−5.1	−1.5
Brukere[c] (users)	467	77	50	.87**	.54	3.5	2.3
Borgere[c] (citizens)	353	−12	−28[d]	.20	−0.61	0.3	−2.2
Jeg OR meg (1 OR me)	25,412	55	15	.98**	.96**	1.8	1.9
Vi OR oss (we OR us)	35,341	16	14	.52**	.95**	0.4	1.6
Likhet[b] (equality)	1,226	−17	−15	−0.92**	−0.19	−1.2	−0.1
Rettferdighet[b] (justice)	249	−32	−12	−0.81**	−0.27	−1.4	−0.7

* Significant at .05 level; ** significant at .01 level

[a]The registration and retrieval procedures of this electronic media archive have been revised/improved several times since the present research commenced in 2002. Moreover, the "rules" for what is included/not included in the archive has varied, for example, according to authors' copyright. Therefore, over time, searches have produced marginally differing results for some search words. However, the overall developmental patterns have been the same

[b]Means that the word string is searched truncated

[c]"Brukere" (users) and "borgere" (citizens) had to be searched in plural to avoid other meanings of the words

[d]Larger increase/decrease in 1999–2008 than 1984–2008 indicates a nonlinear development.

As a consequence of the reported changes, it is also reasonable to expect that the traditional universalistic principle of equality within the Norwegian society, that all citizens have the same value, will also be under attack; social differences will increasingly be accepted. From 1984 through 2008, the frequency of the usage of the word "*likhet*" (equality) is reduced by 17%: a significantly negative correlation with linear time, with an EMAC of −1.2%. The usage of "*rettferdighet*" (justice), moreover, is reduced by 32%: a significantly negative correlation with linear time and an EMAC of −1.4%.

Taken together, the developmental patterns of the various words demonstrate how the currently globalizing ideology with its excessive individualist values and goals is increasingly taking control over the Norwegian language. What about Ghana and the Czech Republic? Do we find the same developmental trends?

Ghana (1999–2008)

Developmental changes over time for the various words in the Ghanaian context are presented in Table 4.2.[9] As can be seen, there is a marked increase of newspaper articles containing words associated with individualism. Number of articles containing "rights" increased by formidable 160%: "I" by 120% and "users" by 42% during this 10-year period. However, at the same time, also the usage of words associated with communality and communal values increased markedly in Ghana. Notably, number of newspaper articles containing "citizens" increased by 140%. Moreover, the usage of "solidarity" and "common" increased by 32% and 34%, respectively. "Equality" and "justice" increased by 77% and 33%, respectively.

It is noticeable that during this relative short period of 10 years, the developmental patterns for a majority of the words correlate significantly with linear time (see Table 4.2). This indicates stable and enduring processes of change. Moreover, the relative strengths of the ongoing changes in Ghana are underlined by high estimated mean annual changes (EMAC): for 11 out of 13 search words, EMAC is higher than 3%.

The Czech Republic

Developmental changes over time for the various words in the Czech context are presented in Table 4.3. As can be seen, for two of the theoretically most central search phrases associated with individualism, "I OR me" and "users," there is only

---

[9] Even though we have data for Ghana back to 1997, here we present data from 1999 only. The reason being that in the Czech Republic, we have data from 1999 only, and in a longitudinal perspective, the difference between 1997 and 1999 is so little that we prefer to have data for identical periods for the two countries. In Table 4.1, Norwegian data for the same period is presented together with data covering the whole period 1984–2008.

Table 4.2 The search words used in the longitudinal (1999–2008) analysis in the Ghanaian society with number of articles observed in 2008, percentage increase/decrease since 1999, correlations (Pearson's r) with linear time (year), and estimated mean annual change (EMAC) for each search word

Search word	Adjusted no. occurrences in 2008	Percent increase/decrease since 1999	Correlation with linear time (year)	Estimated mean annual change (EMAC) (in %)
Rights[a]	821	160	.87**	7.0
Duty	516	14	.06	0.2
Responsibility	671	73	.96**	6.3
Common	859	34	.85**	4.5
Solidarity	93	32	.46	3.3
Cohesion	80	94	.66*	6.5
Belongingness	3	–[b]	.84	20.8
Users[c]	202	42	.52	3.9
Citizens	877	140	.92**	7.9
I[d]	1,806	120	.90**	7.1
We	1,571	95	.84**	6.4
Equality	125	77	.80**	12.5
Justice	1,006	33	.26	1.4

* Significant at .05 level; ** significant at .01 level

[a]"Rights" had to be searched in plural to avoid the meaning of "right" as opposite to left

[b]No observations in 1999

[c]"Users" and "citizens" were searched in plural because the Norwegian "brukere," and "borgere" had to be searched in plural to avoid other meanings of the words

minor increase in usage. However, the usage of the word "rights" decreases markedly by 26%. For the words referring to communality and communal values, there is also a rather mixed pattern. The usage of the majority of the words associated with communal values decreases; for example, "solidarity" decreases by 58%, "responsibility" by 23%, "common" by 17%, and "justice" by 15%. On the other hand, the usage of "cohesion" increases markedly by 59%. Finally, the usage of "citizens" and "equality" did not change at all. Thus, for words associated with individualism as well as for words associated with communal values, we find differential developmental trends in the Czech Republic. For half of the words (6 of 13), the developmental trends correlate significantly with linear time (see Table 4.3).

Norway, Ghana, and the Czech Republic: Comparisons for the Period 1999–2008

Different periods of time (25 years in Norway vs. 10 years in the Czech Republic and Ghana) render comparisons somewhat tentative. Therefore, in Table 4.4, we have excluded major parts of the Norwegian data and present developmental parameters for the years 1999–2008 only for all three countries. However, before comparing the

Table 4.3 The search words used in the longitudinal (1999–2008) analysis in the Czech society with number of articles observed in 2008, percentage increase/decrease since 1999, correlations (Pearson's r) with linear time (year), and estimated mean annual change (EMAC) for each search word

Search word	Adjusted no. occurrences in 2008	Percent increase/decrease since 1999	Correlation with linear time (year)	Estimated mean annual change (EMAC) (in %)
Rights[a]	6,270	−26	−0.79**	−4.1
Duty[b]	3,013	−16	−0.65*	−2.2
Responsibility[c]	2,167	−23	−0.80**	−3.3
Common[d]	6,389	−17	−0.68*	−2.5
Solidarity[e]	299	−58	−0.87**	−10.0
Cohesion[f]	240	59	.75*	5.8
Belongingness[g]	81	−22	−0.58	−4.6
User[h]	816	6	−0.25	−0.5
Citizen[i]	4,572	1	−0.45	−0.9
I or me[j]	35,259	7	.55	1.4
We or us[k]	45,963	−9	−0.38	−0.9
Equality[l]	214	−1	−0.13	−0.9
Justice[m]	1,002	−15	−0.60	−2.0

* Significant at .05 level; ** significant at .01 level
[a]Searched as: právo OR práva OR právu OR právem OR práv OR právům OR právech OR právy
[b]Searched as: povinnost OR povinnosti OR povinností OR povinnostem OR povinnostech OR povinnostmi
[c]Searched as: zodpovědnost OR zodpovědnosti OR zodpovědností OR zodpovědnostem OR zodpovědnostech OR zodpovědnostmi OR odpovědnost OR odpovědnosti OR odpovědností OR odpovědnostem OR odpovědnostech OR odpovědnostmi
[d]Searched as: společný OR společného OR společnému OR společném OR společným OR společná OR společné OR společnou OR společní OR společných OR společnými OR sdílený OR sdíleného OR sdílenému OR sdíleném OR sdíleným OR sdílená OR sdílené OR sdílenou OR sdílení OR sdílených OR sdílenými
[e]Searched as: solidarita OR solidarity OR solidaritě OR solidaritu OR solidarito OR solidaritou OR solidarity OR solidarit OR solidaritám OR solidaritách OR solidaritami
[f]Searched as: soudržnost OR soudržnosti OR soudržností OR soudržnostem OR soudržnostech OR soudržnostmi
[g]Searched as sunálezitost
[h]Searched as: uživatelé OR uživatelů OR uživatelům OR uživatele OR uživatelích OR uživateli OR konzumenti OR konzumentů OR konzumentům OR konzumenty OR konzumentech
[i]Searched as: občané OR občanů OR občanům OR občany OR občanech
[j]Searched as: já OR mě OR mne OR mi OR mně OR mnou
[k]Searched as: my OR nás OR nám OR námi
[l]Searched as: rovnost OR rovnosti OR rovností OR rovnostem OR rovnostech OR rovnostmi
[m]Searched as: spravedlnost OR spravedlnosti OR spravedlností OR spravedlnostem OR spravedlnostech OR spravedlnostmi

three societies across the past decade (1999–2008), it is relevant briefly to comment upon the historical (1984 onward) analyses in Norway. The above-described changes toward strong individualism and weakened communal values in Norway were particularly salient during the late 1980s and throughout the 1990s. For example, "solidaritet" (solidarity) and "samhold" (cohesion) decreased by 43% and 48%,

Table 4.4 Comparison of changes over time in Norway, Ghana, and the Czech Republic during the decade 1999–2008

| | Percent increase/decrease since 1999 | | |
Search word[a]	Norway	Ghana	The Czech Republic
Rights	18	160	−26
Duty	−11	14	−16
Responsibility	−5	73	−23
Common	−2	34	−17
Solidarity	−5	32	−58
Cohesion	−34	94	59
Users	50	42	6
Citizens	−28	140	1
I or me[b]	15	120	7
We or us[c]	14	95	−9
Equality	−15	77	−1
Justice	−12	33	−15

[a]Exact search string for the Norwegian variant of each search word is found in Table 4.1, of the Ghanaian search words in Table 4.2, and of the Czech search words in Table 4.3

[b]Searched as "jeg" OR "meg"' (I OR me) in Norwegian. Searched as "I am" and "I was" in Ghanaian; results presented here are mean values for the two searches. Searched as: já OR mě OR mne OR mi OR mně OR mnou in Czech

[c]Searched as "vi OR oss" (we OR us) in Norwegian. Searched as "we are" and "we were" in Ghanaian; results presented here are mean values for the two searches. Searched as: my OR nás OR nám OR námi in Czech

respectively, from 1990 to 2000, whereas "rettighet" (rights) increased by 17% and "brukere" (users) by formidable 131%. Our analyses indicate that influences in the Norwegian society by globalizing neoliberalism peaked in the early 2000s (cf., also Nafstad et al. 2007, 2009a, b). Observing relative small changes in percentage (Table 4.4), fewer significant correlations with linear time, and smaller EMACs (Tables 4.1, 4.2, and 4.3) in Norway than in the other two societies across the past decade, it is reasonable to assume that globalizing neoliberalism has imbued the Western Norwegian welfare society years before the Ghanaian and Czech societies.

As can be seen in Table 4.4, merely two words demonstrate the same developmental pattern, either increase or decrease in usage, across all three countries. It testifies to the massive global influence of neoliberalism with its strong individualism that the two words, which both demonstrate increasing usage across all the three differential countries, are "I OR me" and "user."

Thus, Norway demonstrates the developmental pattern that we would expect in our era of globalizing neoliberalism: Words referring to individualism increase, whereas words referring to communal values decrease. Characteristic to Ghana is that the individualist as well as the communal words increases markedly in usage. Regarding the consistent and marked increase in usage of communal words, Ghana deviates from both of the two European countries in which usage of communal words decreases. The Czech Republic demonstrate by far the most mixed developmental pattern; whereas the vast majority of the communal words decrease as in the other European country, Norway, one communal word, "cohesion," increases by formidable 59%. Similarly, one of the most individualist words, "rights," does not follow the general trend of individualist words in the Czech Republic and Norway but decreases by a marked 26%.

Limitations of the Present Study

The methodology adopted in the present study has been developed and refined within the Norwegian context for more than a decade (Nafstad 2002; Nafstad et al. 2006, 2007, 2009a, b, c; Rand-Hendriksen 2008). The present study shows that the methodology is promising with regard to exposing culturally different developmental trends as well. However, in future studies, efforts should be taken to elaborate the search systems and the electronic databases in the actual countries (in this case Ghana and the Czech Republic).

Another critical objection could be that we have presented developmental trends of too few words to warrant justifiable interpretations. In order to conclude about the influence of globalizing neoliberalist ideology with its excessive individualism upon language, a greater number of words should be analyzed, thus improving the validity of the description. However, we have, as argued, attempted to select a variety of words representing core aspects of individualist and communal values, respectively. How many words should be included in the analysis is a matter of judgment. We believe that by combining the selected search words, we have offered a useful description of the most salient and relevant ideological shifts across the past years.

Conclusion

The current globalized culture has privileged the ideology of excessive individualism and consumerism. Contending that civic virtues are fundamental for well-being, that human beings are prosocial, and that a good life comprises solidarity and community, we have investigated the interplay between the currently globalized ideology and local ideologies in three different societies. Our parallel longitudinal analyses of changes in language usage in Ghana, Norway, and the Czech Republic demonstrate how local cultures and the forces of globalization merge and shape the resultant ideologies in the public discourse very differently: In all three societies, the usage of words signaling individualism increase. With regard to words signaling communal values, however, the developmental trends differ completely. Whereas the usage of such words decreases in the two European societies, the usage increases markedly in West African Ghana. Finally, developmental trends in the Czech Republic are more mixed than in the other two societies, most probably reflecting the dramatic changes of ideologies this country has undergone after the Iron Curtain was lifted. Thus, the Czech Republic is currently obviously struggling to find a balance between individualist and communal values.

As Delle Fave, Massimini, and Bassi (2011) contend, socio-cultural information, norms, and values undergo dynamic processes of change across time. Currently, late capitalist free-market ideology is spreading across the globe, influencing and changing basic ideologies or value systems within societies around the world. However, every nation has its own economic, political, cultural, and social history which makes each nation negotiate, merge with, and implement the globalized ideologies in unique ways. We have previously argued (Nafstad et al. 2009b) that as a consequence of this complex interplay, positive psychology should continually be attentive to the situation and development of local ideology discourses. Such ideology discourses represent important socio-cultural information; they represent meaning systems, ideals, values, and norms in society and carry tremendous influences on the lives of people as they shape people's belief systems about the good life, well-being, and how to navigate between considerations of their own individual needs and the happiness and the well-being of others and society.

References

Agnew, H. L. (2008). *Češi a země Koruny české*. [Czechs and the lands of the Bohemian Crown]. Praha: Academia.

Akotia, C. S., & Barimah, K. B. (2007). History of community psychology in Ghana. In S. M. Reich, M. Riemer, I. Prilleltensky, & M. Montero (Eds.), *International community psychology. History and theories* (pp. 407–414). New York: Springer.

Akotia, C. S., & Olowu, A. (2000). *Toward an African-centered psychology: Voices of continental African Psychologists*. Paper presented at the 32nd convention of the Association of Black Psychologists, August 2000.

Arnett, J. J. (2002). The psychology of globalization. *American Psychologist, 57*, 774–783.

Aryeetey, E., Harrigan, J., & Nissanke, M. (2000). *Economic reforms in Ghana: The miracle and the mirage*. Trenton: Africa World Press.

Bakhtin, M. M. (1952/1986). *Speech genres and other late essays*. Austin: University of Texas Press.

Batson, C. D. (1991). *The altruism question. Toward a social-psychological answer*. Hillsdale: Lawrence Erlbaum.

Bauman, Z. (2000). *Liquid modernity*. Cambridge: Polity Press.

Billig, M. (1997). Discursive, rhetorical, and ideological messages. In C. McGarty & S. A. Haslam (Eds.), *The message of social psychology* (pp. 36–53). Oxford: Basil Blackwell.

Blakar, R. M. (1973/2006). *Språk er makt*. Oslo: Pax.

Blakar, R. M. (1979). Language as a means of social power. Theoretical-empirical explorations of language and language use as embedded in a social matrix. In J. L. Mey (Ed.), *Pragmalinguistics. Theory and practice* (pp. 131–169). The Hague: Mouton Publishers.

Carlquist, E., Nafstad, H. E., & Blakar, R. M. (2007). Community psychology in a traditional Scandinavian welfare society: The case of Norway. In S. Reich, M. Riemer, I. Prilleltensky, & M. Montero (Eds.), *International community psychology: History and theories* (pp. 282–298). New York: Springer.

Chryssochoou, X. (2004). *Cultural diversity. Its social psychology*. Oxford: Blackwell.

Delle Fave, A., Massimini, F., & Bassi, M. (2011). *Psychological selection and optimal experience across cultures*. Dordrecht: Springer.

Giddens, A. (1991). *Modernity and self-identity: Self and society in the late modern age*. Cambridge: Polity Press.

Hermans, H. J. M., & Kempen, H. J. G. (1998). Moving cultures. The perilous problems of cultural dichotomies in a globalizing society. *American Psychologist, 53*, 1111–1120.

Hoffman, M. L. (1975). Developmental synthesis of affect and cognition and its implications for altruistic motivation. *Developmental Psychology, 11*, 607–622.

Hoffman, M. L. (2000). *Empathy and moral development. Implications for caring and justice*. Cambridge: Cambridge University Press.

Hofstede, G. (1991). *Cultures and organizations: Software in the mind*. London: McGraw-Hill.

Kroskrity, P. V. (Ed.). (2000). *Regimes of language. Ideologies, polities, and identities*. Santa Fe: School of American Research Press.

Lyons, J. (1968). *An introduction to theoretical linguistics*. Cambridge: Cambridge University Press.

Mutz, D. C. (1998). *Impersonal influence. How perceptions of mass collectives affect political attitudes*. Cambridge: Cambridge University Press.

Nafstad, H. E. (2002). The neo-liberal ideology and the self-interest paradigm as resistance to change. *Radical Psychology, 3*, 3–21.

Nafstad, H. E. (2005). Assumptions and values in the production of knowledge: Towards an area ethics of psychology and the social sciences. In S. Robinson & C. Katulushi (Eds.), *Values in higher education* (pp. 150–158). Vale of Glamorgan: Aureus Publishing.

Nafstad, H. E., Carlquist, E., Aasen, I. S., & Blakar, R. M. (2006). Assumptions in psychology and ideological shifts in society: A challenge for positive psychology. In A. Delle Fave (Ed.), *Dimensions of well-being. Research and interventions* (pp. 512–528). Milano: Franco Angeli.

Nafstad, H. E., Blakar, R. M., Carlquist, E., Phelps, J. M., & Rand-Hendriksen, K. (2007). Societal ideology and power: The influence of current neo-liberalism. *Journal of Community and Applied Social Psychology, 17*, 313–327.

Nafstad, H. E., Blakar, R. M., Carlquist, E., Phelps, J. M., & Rand-Hendriksen, K. (2009a). Globalization, neo-liberalism and community psychology. *American Journal of Community Psychology, 43*, 162–175.

Nafstad, H. E., Blakar, R. M., Botchway, A., & Rand-Hendriksen, K. (2009b). Globalization, ideologies and well-being: A study of a West-African and a North-European society. *The Journal of Positive Psychology, 4*, 305–315.

Nafstad, H. E., Blakar, R. M., & Rand-Hendriksen, K. (2009c). The spirit of society and the virtue of gratitude: Shifting societal ideologies of gratitude. In T. Freire (Ed.), *Understanding positive life. Research and practice on positive psychology* (pp. 291–312). Lisboa: Climepsi Editores.

Nafstad, H. E., Carlquist, E., & Blakar, R. M. (2012). Towards a psychology for a humankind and a planet under multiple threats: A social psychology of ideology. In J. P. Valentim (Ed.). *Societal approaches in social psychology*. Bern: Peter Lang Publishing.

Pennebaker, J. W., Mehl, M. R., & Niederhoffer, K. G. (2003). Psychological aspects of natural language use: Our words, our selves. *Annual Review of Psychology, 54*, 547–577.

Peterson, C., & Seligman, M. E. P. (2004). *Character strengths and virtues: A handbook and classification*. New York: Oxford University Press.

Rand-Hendriksen, K. (2008). *Ideological changes measured through changes in language: Development, description and preliminary validation of a new archival method*. Master thesis, University of Oslo, Oslo.

Rommetveit, R. (1968). *Words, meanings and messages*. New York: Academic.

Rommetveit, R., & Blakar, R. M. (1979). *Studies of language, thought and verbal communication*. London: Academic.

Ryan, R. M., Chirkov, V. I., Little, T. D., Sheldon, K. M., Timoshina, E., & Deci, E. L. (1999). The American dream in Russia: Extrinsic aspirations and well-being in two cultures. *Personality and Social Psychology Bulletin, 25*, 1509–1524.

Sampson, E. E. (1981). Cognitive psychology as ideology. *American Psychologist, 36*, 730–743.

Silverstein, M. (1985). Language and the culture of gender: At the intersection of structure, usage and ideology. In E. Mertz & R. J. Parmentier (Eds.), *Semiotic mediation: Sociocultural and psychological perspectives* (pp. 219–259). Orlando: Academic.

Skrbis, Z., Kendall, G., & Woodward, I. (2004). Locating cosmopolitanism. Between humanist ideal and grounded social theory. *Theory, Culture & Society, 21*, 115–136.

Stiglitz, J. E. (2002). *Globalization and its discontents*. New York: W.W. Norton.

Švejnar, J., & Hvížďala, K. (2008). *Kam kráčíš, Česko?* [Where do you go, Czechia?] Praha: Rybka Publishers.

Tashakkori, A., & Teddlie, C. (1998). *Mixed methodology. Combining qualitative and quantitative approaches*. London: Sage Publications.

Triandis, H. C. (1990). Cross-cultural studies of individualism and collectivism. In J. Berman (Ed.), *Nebraska symposium on motivation, 1989* (pp. 41–133). Lincoln: University of Nebraska.

Triandis, H. C. (1995). *Individualism and collectivism*. Boulder: Westview Press.

Triandis, H. C., & Trafimow, D. (2001). Cross-national prevalence of collectivism. In C. Sedikides & M. B. Brewer (Eds.), *Individual self, relational self, collective self* (pp. 259–276). Philadelphia: Psychology Press.

van Dijk, T. A. (1998). *Ideology: A multidisciplinary approach*. London: Sage.

Wilson, R. W. (1992). *Compliance ideologies. Rethinking political culture*. New York: Cambridge University Press.

Chapter 5
The Relation of Basic Psychological Needs, Intrinsic and Extrinsic Life Goals, and Collectivism with Subjective Well-Being: A Case in Macedonia

Ognen Spasovski

Introduction

In developed countries, there is a well-established model which suggests that subjective well-being is a direct function of basic psychological needs satisfaction, where realization of intrinsic life goals is beneficial, but pursuing extrinsic life goals on the contrary thwarts such satisfaction (Deci and Ryan 1991; Ryan and Deci 2001). Could this model be applied to a socioeconomic and cultural context such as the Macedonian? Macedonia is an ex-communist country in development, still struggling with devastating transition. Through many decades in the communistic past, there was no obvious social stratification, and most people when compared to others did not perceive significant social differences. Society was supposed to provide social security and well-being to all, and it was a common behavior that the state (institutions) plan many significant life areas. In such conditions, individual initiative was becoming inhibited, and the sense of responsibility for personal choices was shared with the state. During the transition period, rapid changes happened. In short time, some people became rich, and some obtained high status and became very famous. Other people became very poor. Many felt miserable. The state was not providing social security and equality any more. Everything became accessible if one succeeds to achieve it. However, at the same time, the success criteria changed. People were forced to pursue new goals in the pursuit of a new life. They were exposed to changed values. Individualistic values were becoming more and more salient. This phenomenon is very significant knowing that according to recent findings, Macedonian society is dominantly oriented toward collectivistic values (Kenig 2006).

O. Spasovski, Ph.D. (✉)
Department of Psychology, Faculty of Philosophy, Ss Cyril and Methodius University
in Skopje, Blvd Krste Misirkov bb, 1000 Skopje, Republic of Macedonia
e-mail: ognen@fzf.ukim.edu.mk; ognen@sas.upenn.edu

H.H. Knoop and A. Delle Fave (eds.), *Well-Being and Cultures: Perspectives
from Positive Psychology*, Cross-Cultural Advancements in Positive Psychology 3,
DOI 10.1007/978-94-007-4611-4_5, © Springer Science+Business Media Dordrecht 2013

This study aims to test the model in such context. There are two starting points. First, the views of Self-Determination Theory (Deci and Ryan 1991; Ryan and Deci 2001) that subjective well-being is a direct function of the satisfaction of basic psychological needs, which is closely related with the pursuing and realization of intrinsic life goals. Second, we have the specific Macedonian socioeconomic and cultural context. Starting from these propositions, the *problem of this research* is to explore whether the subjective well-being is related to the basic psychological needs, aspirations toward intrinsic and extrinsic life goals, and orientation toward collectivism at individual level. Concerning cultural specifics, it was *hypothesized* that subjective well-being is positively related with the satisfaction of basic psychological needs, with the aspiration for both intrinsic and extrinsic life goals, as well as with the orientation toward collectivism.

Defining Concepts

Subjective well-being is understood as optimal psychological functioning, manifested through positive feeling toward oneself and our own life. Subjective well-being is a personal experience resulting from self-evaluation of life in general – what is significantly based on the evaluation of our realized desires and valued things that will make our life fulfilled and pleasant. Hence, subjective well-being is operationally defined as frequently experiencing satisfaction with life and pleasant emotions and only rarely unpleasant emotions (Diener et al. 1997; Diener and Lucas 2000; Oishi and Diener 2001; Schimmack et al. 2004).

Basic psychological needs are internal conditions necessary for continuous psychic development, integrity, and well-being. They energize the person, and their satisfaction contributes to psychic health and well-being, while thwarting is followed by ill-being (Baumeister and Leary 1995; Deci and Ryan 2000; Ryan and Deci 2000). When satisfied, they do not motivate; when unsatisfied, they urge the organism and then needs become motives (Smith 1992). It is conceptualized that there are three basic psychological needs: a need for autonomy, for competence, and for relatedness.

Intrinsic and extrinsic life goals: In the literature related to this topic, differentiation between intrinsic and extrinsic motivation has long history. Life goals are considered as specific motivational projections or outcomes which direct the person through life. They are conscious and differ from biological needs. They are based on values, but are narrower constructs (Schmuck and Sheldon 2001). References related to Self-Determination Theory (SDT) have only recently made a distinction between intrinsic goal contents and extrinsic goal contents (Kasser and Ryan 1993, 1996, 2001; Sheldon and Kasser 1995, 2001; Wrosch et al. 2007). Kasser and Ryan (1996) defined intrinsic goals, such as those for personal growth, emotional intimacy/meaningful relationships, and community contribution/involvement, as ones that are inherently rewarding to pursue, presumably because they directly satisfy innate psychological needs such as belongingness (Baumeister and Leary 1995; Baumeister 1999), effectance (White 1959), and personal causation (De Charms 1968). Those needs in SDT are defined as relatedness, competence, and autonomy (Deci and Ryan 2000). Extrinsic life goals are those for financial success (material wealth), fame/status, and image; pursuing such goals is not inherently rewarding.

Collectivism is understood as devotion to the values, norms, standards, and criteria of the group and closer community. It supposes integration in cohesive groups which procure protection. Collectivism means preference of group work instead of individual work, as well as tendency to maintain the group harmony. Hofstede compares individualism to collectivism as valuing individual freedom despite group harmony (Kenig 2006). According to the latest findings, collectivistic orientation prevails in the Republic of Macedonia (Kenig 2006).

Method

Participants and Procedure

The study used a convenient sample of 242 participants, second year undergraduates at the State University in Skopje, R. of Macedonia. They came from three different study fields: natural sciences, social sciences, and technical studies. Table 5.1 shows the structure with regard to the study program and sex/gender. Their average age is 20.6 years, ranging from 19 to 26. Regarding their ethnicity, 92% are ethnic Macedonians, 3.3% belong to the community of ethnic Albanians in Macedonia, 2.1% are Vlachs, and 2.7% are other nationalities. All the tests were administered on one occasion, rotating the order of tests in every study group. Testing was realized during their regular classes, participants receiving a credit for participation as incentive.

Measures

Subjective well-being: Many authors referred to life satisfaction and positive affect, the inverse of negative affect, as the primary components of subjective well-being. A composite subjective well-being index could be created from these three components (Sheldon and Elliot 1999; Reis et al. 2000) after their standardization. To assess positive and negative affect, participants were tested on Positive and Negative Affect

Table 5.1 Structure of the sample with regard to study field and gender

Study group	Female	Male	Total
Technical studies	50	40	90
Social studies	60	23	83
Natural studies	41	28	69
Total	151	91	*242*

Schedule (PANAS) (Watson and Clark 1994). Having 20 emotion adjectives, 10 positive and 10 negative, participants indicated the extent to which they generally feel each way using a 1 (*not at all*) to 5 (*very much*) scale. According to the authors and confirmed in other studies (Brown and Marshall 2001), the instrument has a solid reliability ($\alpha=.87$ for positive emotions and $\alpha=.85$ for negative emotions). Checked on the data of this study, reliability is $\alpha=.71$ for positive emotions and $\alpha=.82$ for negative emotions. For the other component, the Satisfaction With Life Scale (SWLS) (Diener et al. 1985) was administered, which contains five statements such as "In most ways my life is close to my ideal." Participants indicated their agreement with each item in general using a 7-point scale. The instrument has a satisfactory reliability (α between .80 and .87). The reliability coefficient obtained in this research is .81.

Basic psychological needs: General Need Satisfaction Scale (Ilardi et al. 1993) measures the level of satisfaction of three basic psychological needs, for competence, autonomy, and relatedness. Accordingly, it consists of three subscales with 21 items ($\alpha=.89$). Correlations between subscales have values from .61 to .66. Participants responded on a scale from 1 (meaning absolutely disagree) to 7 (absolutely agree/true). The coefficient of reliability is $\alpha=.71$; calculated on data from this study, it is $\alpha=.79$.

Intrinsic and extrinsic life goals: Aspirations Index (Kasser and Ryan 1993, 1996) measures level of aspiration toward intrinsic or extrinsic motivation. It has seven subscales for all six intrinsic and extrinsic life goals already mentioned, plus orientation toward health, which is neither intrinsic nor extrinsic. That is the reason why this health subscale is not included in the study. Alpha coefficient of reliability is between .71 and .83 (Kasser and Ryan 1996; Frost and Frost 2000), and calculated on data from this study, it is 0.9.

Collectivism: Yamaguchi Collectivism Scale (adopted by Kenig 2006) is used. The scale has 10 items. Participants indicate their agreement from 1 (absolutely disagree) to 7 (absolutely agree). Crombach's alpha coefficient is $\alpha=.68$, and calculated on data from this study, it is $\alpha=.616$.

Results

The results from the *correlation analysis* show that subjective well-being significantly and highly correlates with the main motivational variables, basic psychological needs, and life goals (Table 5.2). An important finding is the high correlation between subjective well-being and extrinsic life goals ($r=0.31; p<.001$). The results further show that subjective well-being correlates moderately yet significantly with the orientation toward collectivism.

In Table 5.3, the results from the correlation analysis between subjective well-being and all of the separate basic psychological needs are given. It can be seen that the correlation is very high with all of the needs, with coefficients between .42 and .50.

Table 5.2 Matrix of correlations between subjective well-being and basic psychological needs, life goals, and collectivism

	Subjective well-being	BPN total	Intrinsic LG	Extrinsic LG	Collectivism
Subjective wellbeing	1	.60***	.42***	.31***	.185*
	–	.001	.001	.001	.021
BPN total	–	1	.52***	.29***	.144*
	–	–	.001	.001	.013
Intrinsic LG	–	–	1	.49***	.227**
	–	–	–	.001	.006
Extrinsic LG	–	–	–	1	−.047
	–	–	–	–	.305
Collectivism	–	–	–	–	1
	–	–	–	–	–

Below the values of the correlation in the tables, given are the exact *p* values
BNP basic psychological needs; *LG* life goals
***Correlation is significant at the 0.001 level; **correlation is significant at the 0.01 level; *correlation is significant at the 0.05 level

Table 5.3 Matrix of correlations between subjective well-being and basic psychological needs for autonomy, competence and relatedness, and total

	Subjective well-being	BPN for autonomy	BPN for competence	BPN for relatedness	BPN total
Subjective well-being	1	.50***	.50***	.42***	.60***
	–	.001	.001	.001	.001
BPN for autonomy	–	1	.41***	.52***	.81***
	–	–	.001	.001	.001
BPN for competence	–	–	1	.40***	.76***
	–	–	–	.001	.001
BPN for relatedness	–	–	–	1	.80***
	–	–	–	–	.001
BPN total	–	–	–	–	1
	–	–	–	–	–

Below the values of the correlation in the tables, the exact *p* values are given
***Correlation is significant at the 0.001 level

Table 5.4 shows the results from the analysis of correlation between subjective well-being and all life goals separately. With regard to the relation between subjective well-being to intrinsic goals, it could be seen that the correlation is significant with all of them. The correlation is the highest with the goal for personal growth ($r=.31$; $p < .001$), then with the goal to have and maintain significant relationships ($r=.22$; $p < .01$), and the lowest correlation is with the goal to contribute to the community ($r=.17$; $p < .05$). Regarding the relation between subjective well-being to extrinsic goals, the results show that subjective well-being significantly correlates with the goal to acquire wealth ($r=.21$; $p < .01$) and with the goal for status/fame ($r=.20$; $p < .05$). There is no significant correlation with the goal to take care and maintain the image.

Table 5.4 Matrix of correlations between subjective well-being and all separate intrinsic and extrinsic life goals

	Subjective well-being	Personal growth	Relationships	Contribution community	Material wealth	Status/ fame	Image
Subjective	1	.312***	.220**	.174*	.215**	.197*	.077
well-being	–	.001	.008	.028	.009	.016	.202
Personal growth	–	1	.325***	.339***	.309***	.225**	.249**
	–	–	.001	.001	.001	.007	.003
Relationships	–	–	1	.355**	.155*	.155*	.234**
	–	–	–	.001	.045	.046	.005
Contrib. commun.	–	–	–	1	.345***	.485***	.482***
	–	–	–	–	.001	.001	.001
Material wealth	–	–	–	–	1	.413***	.535***
	–	–	–	–	–	.001	.001
Status/fame	–	–	–	–	–	1	.604***
	–	–	–	–	–	–	.001
Image	–	–	–	–	–	–	1
	–	–	–	–	–	–	–

Below the values of the correlation in the tables, the exact p values are given
***Correlation is significant at the 0.001 level; **correlation is significant at the 0.01 level; *correlation is significant at the 0.05 level

Table 5.5 Results of regression analysis predicting subjective well-being from total scores for basic psychological needs, life goals, and collectivism

Model	R^2 change	Sig.	Beta	Sig.
Step 1	.362	.001		
BPN total			.601	.001
Step 2	.028	.001		
BPN total			.560	.001
Extrinsic LG			.173	.001

Criterion variable: subjective well-being

Regression analysis: Results from the regression analysis (step by step model was used) in Table 5.5 show that when all variables were entered in the analysis as possible predictors (total scores for basic psychological needs, intrinsic and extrinsic life goals, and collectivism), the basic psychological needs (BPN total) ($\beta = .560$, $p < .001$) and extrinsic life goals ($\beta = .173$, $p < .001$) were specified as significant predictors of subjective well-being, and they together explain (in Step 2) 39% of participants' variability in scores on subjective well-being. The analysis excluded all the other variables as nonsignificant predictors of subjective well-being.

Regression analysis was done again separately for all basic psychological needs (Table 5.6) and for all life goals as potential predictors (Table 5.7).

It is evident from Table 5.6 that the model assigns all basic psychological needs as significant predictors, explaining 37.2% of participants' variability in scores on

Table 5.6 Results of regression analysis predicting subjective well-being from basic psychological needs for autonomy, competence, and relatedness

Model	R^2 change	Sig.	Beta	Sig.
Step 1	.254	.001		
Autonomy			.504	.001
Step 2	.106	.001		
Autonomy			.358	.001
Competence			.357	.001
Step 3	.012	.032		
Autonomy			.300	.001
Competence			.328	.001
Relatedness			.133	.032

Criterion variable: subjective well-being

Table 5.7 Results of regression analysis predicting subjective well-being from intrinsic and extrinsic life goals

Model	R^2 change	Sig.	Beta	Sig.
Step 1	.174	.001		
Personal growth			.417	.001
Step 2	.033	.002		
Personal growth			.330	.001
Relationships			.202	.001
Step 3	.024	.007		
Personal growth			.289	.001
Relationships			.193	.002
Status/fame			.161	.007

Criterion variable: subjective well-being

subjective well-being. In addition, Table 5.7 shows that two intrinsic (personal growth and meaningful relationships) and one extrinsic life goal (status/fame) are significant predictors of subjective well-being, explaining 23.1% of variability.

Discussion

Study findings discover some new trends, especially with regard to the role of extrinsic life goals and orientation toward collectivism.

Firstly, as was expected based on previous research, results showed that basic psychological needs and intrinsic goals correlate highly with subjective well-being. These findings are congruent with those of Kasser and Ryan's with regard to life goals (Kasser and Ryan 1993, 1996, 2001), as well as with the findings of many other studies predominantly conducted in the "Western" world (Ryan et al. 1999; Schmuck et al. 2000; Grouzet et al. 2005), but also with the study findings from

Croatia as ex-communistic country (Brdar 2006). Furthermore, the results are congruent with the findings on the relation between the satisfaction of basic psychological needs and subjective well-being (Ryan and Deci 2000; Sheldon and Kasser (1995) VitVis important for the person to choose and develop life goals concordant with the authentic needs and values (Sheldon and Kasser 1995, 2001). This time, confirmation is based on the data obtained from participants from ex-communist developing country.

Very important result is that extrinsic goals also significantly correlate with subjective well-being, which is not congruent with the findings from developed countries. This possibly reveals a different role and mechanism of extrinsic goals with regard to their relation to the basic psychological needs and subjective well-being. As seen from the correlation matrix related to extrinsic goals, subjective well-being correlates the highest with *wealth* (financial success), where coefficient is close to the coefficient for *meaningful relationships* as an intrinsic goal. Subjective well-being also significantly correlates with *fame/status*, but not with *image*.

What could be that role of extrinsic goals in such constellations? One possible explanation is that minimum material goods are a kind of prerequisite for satisfying basic psychological needs and obtaining optimal subjective well-being. Compliant with this result are the findings of Frost and Frost in a comparative study on samples from USA and Romania. In the Romanian sample, the increase of extrinsic aspirations was not followed by the decrease of subjective well-being (Frost and Frost 2000). Veenhoven argues that in some societies, material conditions are very important for subjective well-being, having such reasoning being confirmed in many studies (Veenhoven 2000, 2006; Inglehart and Klingemann 2000; Diener and Suh 2000; Diener and Oishi 2000; Biswas-Diener 2008). Macedonian society is a society of that kind. The possible mechanism is as follows: When the realization of intrinsic life goals is thwarted, having as a consequence that basic psychological needs will probably not be satisfied, the extrinsic aspirations assume a specific role. Processes of realization of extrinsic goals probably compensate for the psychic gap or emptiness from the unsatisfied basic psychological needs and create the least minimum conditions for their satisfaction. Here probably underlies the positive relation between the pursuit of extrinsic goals and subjective well-being. This relation is probably "effective" until extrinsic goals are not more important and aspired than intrinsic goals.

In transitional society with changing values as explained previously, the financial success becomes a significant indicator of someone's capability (experience related to oneself and one's competence, which inevitably influences subjective well-being). As a result, the sense of the satisfaction of basic psychological need for competence becomes influenced by external factors. Among the strongest factors are the amount someone earns and the degree of prestigious status a person has. To have such "criteria" is paradoxical because it seems that many people pursue a set of goals which are unreachable. Today, there are more opportunities and wealth in the world than ever, but the sense of well-being and happiness has not changed significantly. Projections of all material things "needed" by people today could four-fold cover the planet (Schmuck et al. 2000). It is typical for humans to have such expanding demands probably related to the belief that the more we have, the higher the probability for happiness, thus getting a higher status in the community. That way, the process of self-evaluation of personal competence becomes influenced by such external factors, contrary to the belief that (only) internal factors generate happiness. Those results raise the question whether Western models (as Self-Determination Theory) are applicable to societies as Macedonian.

Finally, results from the correlation analysis regarding the *orientation toward collectivism* show significant positive relation to subjective well-being. Here, the explanation is closely connected with the cultural context, or the reality of Macedonian society as predominantly collectivistic. What does this imply on an individual level? One possible interpretation is that the acceptance of collectivistic values in a collectivistic community has an adaptive function for most of the individuals, followed by lesser confrontation with the norms of the community and with the people from our (collectivistic) surrounding. Such experiences probably produce less negative emotions, closer relationships, and greater satisfaction with life.

The regression analysis results gave us significant predictors in three different models. Table 5.5 (with all total scores) underlined basic psychological needs and extrinsic life goals as significant predictors. This could be interpreted in accordance with the hypothesis of the complementary role of extrinsic goals, while the exclusion of intrinsic life goals could be explained by having the same underlying factors with the basic psychological needs. The second model (Table 5.6) gave us all basic psychological needs as significant predictors. The third model (Table 5.7), with all life goals included, gave interesting results. As continuation to the discussion above, regression analysis shows an intriguing result that pursuit and realization of extrinsic life goal for status/fame is a significant predictor of subjective well-being, while the intrinsic life goal for contribution to the community is not! It should be explored further the nature and the role of pursuing the life goal for status. And more important, to explore why contribution to the community is not a desirable goal. What is going on with the society where for the young members, even more students, it is not valuable to make some contribution to the community? Being in the same time more attracted by reaching higher status or to become famous.

Conclusions: Basic psychological needs and intrinsic life goals are positively related with subjective well-being, which was expected. Study results also show that extrinsic life goals are positively and highly related with the subjective well-being. Furthermore, the orientation toward collectivism is positively related with subjective well-being, suggesting that it is beneficial to be collectivist in a collectivistic country.

Limitations: Using instruments created in predominantly individualistic Western cultures in sociocultural context as Macedonian creates certain difficulties in the testing process which limits the findings. In addition, the results could not be generalized to all ethnic communities in Macedonia, especially to Albanian ethnic community as the biggest community after ethnic Macedonians, because participants of Albanian nationality were underrepresented in the sample.

References

Baumeister, R. F. (1999). Introduction. In R. F. Baumeister (Ed.), *The self in social psychology*. Ann Arbor: Taylor & Francis Group.

Baumeister, R. F., & Leary, M. R. (1995). The need to belong: Desire for interpersonal attachments as a fundamental human motivation. *Psychological Bulletin, 117*, 497–529.

Biswas-Diener, R. M. (2008). Material wealth and subjective well-being. In M. Eid & R. J. Larsen (Eds.), *The science of subjective well-being*. London: Guilford Press.

Brdar, I. (2006). Životni ciljevi i dobrobit: je li za sreću važno što želimo? *Društvena istraživanja, 4–5*, 671–691. [Life goals and well-being: Is for happiness important what we want? *Societal Research, 4–5*, 671–691].

Brown, J. D., & Marshall, M. A. (2001). Self-esteem and emotion: Some thoughts about feelings. *Personality and Social Psychology Bulletin, 7*, 575–584.

De Charms, R. (1968). *Personal causation: The internal affective determinants of behavior*. New York: Academic.

Deci, E. L., & Ryan, R. M. (1991). A motivational approach to self: Integration in personality. In R. Dienstbier (Ed.), *Nebraska symposium on motivation* (Perspectives on motivation, Vol. 38, pp. 237–288). Lincoln: University of Nebraska Press.

Deci, E. L., & Ryan, R. M. (2000). The "what" and "why" of goal pursuits: Human needs and the self-determination of behavior. *Psychological Inquiry, 11*, 227–268.

Diener, E., & Lucas, R. E. (2000). Subjective emotional well-being. In M. Lewis & J. M. Haviland (Eds.), *Handbook of emotions* (2nd ed., pp. 325–337). New York: Guilford.

Diener, E., & Oishi, S. (2000). Money and happiness. In E. Diener & E. M. Suh (Eds.), *Culture and subjective well-being* (pp. 185–218). London: The MIT Press.

Diener, E., & Suh, E. M. (2000). Measuring subjective well-being to compare the quality of life of cultures. In E. Diener & E. M. Suh (Eds.), *Culture and subjective well-being*. London: The MIT Press.

Diener, E., Emmons, R. A., Larsen, R. J., & Griffin, S. (1985). The satisfaction with life scale. *Journal of Personality Assessment, 49*, 71–75.

Diener, E., Suh, E., & Oishi, S. (1997). Recent findings on subjective well-being. *Indian Journal of Clinical Psychology, 24*, 25–41.

Frost, K. M., & Frost, J. C. (2000). Romanian and American life aspirations in relation to psychological well-being. *Journal of Cross-Cultural Psychology, 31*, 726–751.

Grouzet, F. M., Kasser, T., Ahuvia, A., Dols, J. M., Kim, Y., Lau, S., Ryan, R. M., Saunders, S., Schmuck, P., & Sheldon, K. M. (2005). The structure of goals across 15 cultures. *Journal of Personality and Social Psychology, 89*, 800–816.

Ilardi, B. C., Leone, D., Kasser, R., & Ryan, R. M. (1993). *General need satisfaction scale*. http://www.psych.rochester.edu/SDT/measures/bpns_scale.php. Accessed 20 Mar 2008.

Inglehart, R., & Klingemann, H.-D. (2000). Genes, culture, democracy and happiness. In E. Diener & E. M. Suh (Eds.), *Culture and subjective well-being* (pp. 165–184). London: The MIT Press.

Kasser, T., & Ryan, R. M. (1993). A dark side of the American dream: Correlates of financial success as a central life aspiration. *Journal of Personality and Social Psychology, 65*, 410–422.

Kasser, T., & Ryan, R. M. (1996). Further examining the American dream: Differential correlates of intrinsic and extrinsic goals. *Personality and Social Psychology Bulletin, 22*, 280–287.

Kasser, T., & Ryan, R. M. (2001). Be careful what you wish for: Optimal functioning and the relative attainment of intrinsic and extrinsic goals. In P. Schmuck & K. M. Sheldon (Eds.), *Life goals and well-being: Towards a positive psychology of human striving* (pp. 116–131). Goetitingen: Hogrefe & Huber.

Kenig, N. (2006). *Hofstedoviot model na dimenzii na kulturata: Možnosti za merenje vo grupen i individualen kontekst*. Neobjavena doktorska disertacija. Filozofski fakultet, Skopje. [*Hofsted's model of dimensions of culture: Possibilities for assessment in group and individual context*. Doctoral dissertation. Faculty of Philosophy, Skopje].

Oishi, S., & Diener, E. (2001). Goals, culture, and subjective well-being. *Personality and Social Psychology Bulletin, 27,* 1674–1682.

Reis, H. T., Sheldon, K. M., Gable, S. L., Roscoe, J., & Ryan, R. M. (2000). Daily well-being: The role of autonomy, competence, and relatedness. *Personality and Social Psychology Bulletin, 26,* 419–435.

Ryan, R. M., & Deci, E. L. (2000). The darker and brighter sides of human existence: Basic psychological needs as a unifying concept. *Psychological Inquiry, 11,* 319–338.

Ryan, R. M., & Deci, E. L. (2001). On happiness and human potentials: A review of research on hedonic and eudaimonic well-being. *Annual Review of Psychology, 52,* 141–166.

Ryan, R. M., Chirkov, V. I., Little, T. D., Sheldon, K. M., Timoshina, E., & Deci, E. L. (1999). The American Dream in Russia: Extrinsic aspirations and well-being in two cultures. *Personality and Social Psychology Bulletin, 25,* 1509–1524.

Schimmack, U., Oishi, S., Furr, M. R., & Funder, D. C. (2004). Personality and life satisfaction: A facet-level analysis. *Personality and Social Psychology Bulletin, 30,* 1062–1075.

Schmuck, P., & Sheldon, K. M. (2001). *Life goals and well-being: Towards a positive psychology of human striving.* Goetingen: Hogrefe & Huber.

Schmuck, P., Kasser, T., & Ryan, R. M. (2000). The relationship of well-being to intrinsic and extrinsic goals in Germany and the U.S. *Social Indicators Research, 50,* 225–241.

Sheldon, K. M., & Kasser, T. (1995). Coherence and congruence: Two aspects of personality integration. *Journal of Personality and Social Psychology, 68,* 531–543.

Sheldon, K. M., & Elliot, A. J. (1999). Goal striving, need-satisfaction, and longitudinal well-being: The Self-Concordance Model. *Journal of Personality and Social Psychology, 76,* 482–497.

Sheldon, K. M., & Kasser, T. (2001). Goals, congruence, and positive well-being: New empirical support. *Journal of Humanistic Psychology, 41*(1), 30–50.

Smith, M. B. (1992). *Values, self and society: Toward a humanist social psychology.* New Brunswick: Transaction Publishers.

Veenhoven, R. (2000). Freedom and happiness: A comparative study in forty-four nations in early 1990s. In E. Diener & E. M. Suh (Eds.), *Culture and subjective well-being* (pp. 257–288). London: The MIT Press.

Veenhoven, R. (2006). *Average happiness in 95 nations 1995–2005.* World Database of Happiness, RankReport 2006–1d, www.worlddatabaseofhappiness.eur.nl. Accessed 15 Apr 2008.

Watson, D., & Clark, L. A. (1994). *The PANAS-X: Manual for the positive and negative affect schedule – expanded from.* Iowa: The University of Iowa.

White, R. W. (1959). Motivation reconsidered: The concept of competence. *Psychological Review, 66,* 297–333.

Wrosch, C., Miller, G. E., Scheier, M. F., & Brun de Pontet, S. (2007). Giving Up on unattainable goals: Benefits for health? *Personality and Social Psychology Bulletin, 33,* 251.

Chapter 6
The Ubiquity of the Character Strengths in African Traditional Religion: A Thematic Analysis

Sahaya G. Selvam and Joanna Collicutt

Introduction

Religious Traditions and the Character Strengths

The catalogue of core virtues and character strengths (Peterson and Seligman 2004), or the "Values in Action" (VIA; Peterson 2006), has become for positive psychology what DSM-IV or ICD-10 has been for psychiatry. Empirical research within positive psychology has been greatly influenced by this "catalogue of sanities".

Virtue in positive psychology (PP) is understood as "any psychological process that enables a person to think and act so as to benefit him- or herself and the society" (McCullough and Snyder 2000: 1). In other words, virtue contributes to subjective, psychological and social well-being. Peterson and Seligman (2004: 13) further suggest that virtues "are universal, perhaps grounded in biology through an evolutionary process that selected for these aspects of excellence as means of solving the important tasks necessary for survival of the species". Virtues are expressed in character strengths. "Character strengths (CS) are the psychological ingredients – processes or mechanisms – that define the virtues. Said another way, they are distinguishable routes to displaying one or another of the virtues" (p. 14). They are different from talents and abilities but composed of a family of positive traits which lead to human flourishing.

S.G. Selvam (✉)
Institute of Youth Ministry, Tangaza College,
Nairobi 15055-00509, Kenya
e-mail: selvam@donbosco.or.tz; S.Selvam@heythropcollege.ac.uk

J. Collicutt
Psychology of Religion, Harris Manchester College, Mansfield Road,
Oxford OX1 3TD, UK
e-mail: joanna.collicutt@hmc.ox.ac.uk

H.H. Knoop and A. Delle Fave (eds.), *Well-Being and Cultures: Perspectives from Positive Psychology*, Cross-Cultural Advancements in Positive Psychology 3, DOI 10.1007/978-94-007-4611-4_6, © Springer Science+Business Media Dordrecht 2013

One of the criteria applied in the original selection of the candidate strengths to the catalogue of the VIA was their ubiquity across cultures and religious traditions (Park and Peterson 2007: 296; Peterson and Seligman 2004: 14–27; Peterson 2006: 29–48). More precisely, this was achieved by examining the philosophical and religious traditions of China (Confucianism and Taoism), South Asia (Buddhism and Hinduism) and the West and Ancient near East (Ancient Greek philosophy, Judaism, Christianity and Islam), looking for the insights each provide for the pleasant, good and engaged life (Dahlsgaard et al. 2005; Peterson and Seligman 2004: 33–52; Snyder and Lopez 2007: 23–50).

Earlier, Haidt (2003: 275) had invited scholars within positive psychology to look "to other cultures and other historical eras for ideas and perspectives on virtue and the good life". He supposed that world religions hold a great promise of a "highly developed and articulated visions of virtues, practices and feelings, some of which may even be useful in a modern secular society". In a similar vein, Maltby and Hill (2008) see religion as a fertile ground for positive psychologists to study systematically the "common denominators" of virtues and character strengths. There have been other similar efforts in facilitating a dialogue between positive psychology and various religious traditions, either in support, or in critique, of positive psychology and its constructs (Chu and Diener 2009; Delle Fave and Bassi 2009a; Sundararajan 2005; Joseph et al. 2006; Watts et al. 2006; Vitz 2005; Zagano and Gillespie 2006).

In all these discussions, reference to African traditional religion (ATR) is minimal. Even in research works carried out in South Africa (see Coetzee and Viviers 2007; Eloff 2008) ATR gets no mention. Worthy of mention here, though, is the work by Biswas-Diener (2006) that evaluates the existence, importance and desirability of character strengths across cultures. This study included a sample ($n = 123$) of the Kenyan Maasai. Yet another web-based study on character strengths (Nansook et al. 2006) drew data from 54 nations, including four African countries. The aim of the present qualitative study was to supplement this ongoing discussion on the ubiquity of character strengths across cultures and religious traditions with input from cultural and religious traditions of Africa.

African Traditional Religion

Politically, the adjective "African" is often used to refer to the whole continent of Africa as it is understood within the African Union (as also some historians do: see Mazrui 1986: 26–29). On account of its diversities, this geographical identity is hardly appropriate while speaking about African cultures and religions. Given the prevalence of the Mediterranean world view in countries that lie to the north of the Sahara, cultural anthropologists prefer to speak of the sub-Saharan Africa as a cultural locus (see Shillington 2005). Despite their own linguistic, political and historical variations, certain commonalities of culture and world view are identifiable, particularly within the beliefs and practices of the traditional religions (Beugré and Offodile 2001; Selvam 2008).

Scholars have often referred to traditional religions as "primitive" (Tylor 1871/1958; see also P'Bitek 1970). This term generally carried a pejorative meaning. However, looked at positively, the term "primitive" could imply that these religions and practices preserve the early stages of human religious consciousness and its expressions. According to this understanding, the study of "indigenous religions" (Cox 2007) offers us a possibility of encountering the human psyche in its primeval form (Lowie 1924). Thus, the study of African religions could open a window to the world view and the psyche of not only the African peoples but of humanity itself.

Some anthropologists like Mbiti (1969) prefer to speak of "religions" in the plural, because there are about 1,000 ethnic groups in Africa and each has its own cultural peculiarities while sharing certain commonality in the religious system. Therefore, African traditional religion does not refer to a monolithic institution. On the other hand, on account of the commonalities present, other scholars refer to African religion in the singular (Magesa 1998) or to African traditional religion (Idowu 1973; Shorter 1975). While recognising the issue of religious diversity, it can be argued that the commonalities outweigh the differences, and in this article, the singular form is maintained on the grounds of commonalities suggested by Magesa (1998).

ATR can be described as a collection of beliefs, codes and cults that encapsulate the primeval experiences and expressions of the African peoples in their search for the sacred. Here, belief is understood as a set of possible explanations for the mysteries of the origin and nature of the world and of humans and how humans may interact with the empirical world of objects, people and the non-empirical world of spirit(s). Beliefs in ATR are not seen in dogmas and doctrines. They are to be recognised in oral traditions that include myths, riddles, aphorisms and the cult itself. Code is the set of taboos and casuistry that ensure the preservation and the continuity of human life and its relation to the sacred (see Magesa 1998; Nkemnkia 1999). Cult contains the various expressions of the relationship between the living and the sacred that includes the living dead (the ancestors) and the yet unborn. From the psychological perspective, cult also plays an important role in accompanying individuals in negotiating the various stages of lifespan development.

For all the variety that is undeniable in the religious expressions found in sub-Saharan Africa, one commonality that is crucial, even to this essay, is that in ATR there is no separation of the sacred from the profane (Durkheim 1915; Evans-Pritchard 1965), and because of this, scholars have often spoken about African philosophy and culture in conjunction with African religion (Magesa 1998; Mbiti 1969; Taylor 1963). This justifies the use of anthropological data for the present study, which focuses on the ubiquity of character strengths in African traditional religion.

Research Questions

The objective of this study was to explore the presence and nature of the core virtues and character strengths of positive psychology in ATR. This qualitative study began with two generic research questions:

(a) Can the core virtues of PP be consistently discerned within a sample of textual anthropological data on ATR?
(b) How can the six core virtues of positive psychology be understood within the discourse of ATR while rendering ATR in the contemporary lexical and thematic discourse of PP?

Method

Data Set

The data used for this qualitative analysis was a set of raw data in textual form previously collected and published by the Maryknoll Institute of African Studies (MIAS) in Nairobi, Kenya (Kirwen 2008). MIAS offers graduate degrees in anthropology and African studies. Based on field research carried out for over 17 years, the institute has identified 35 domains in cultural studies. These domains are further delineated into four cycles, namely, (1) individual life cycle, (2) family and interpersonal relationships cycle, (3) community and communal activities cycle and (4) religious rituals cycle (Kirwen 2008). The present study used the data available under the first cycle, which comprised ten domains (Table 6.1).

The present data were collected in English from graduate students ($N=75$) during the MIAS academic programmes, between January and August 2003. The students were asked to reflect on some open questions (Table 6.1) and briefly write out the meanings of cultural domains within their personal lives and that of the cultures from which they come. The questions were answered also by non-African students; their responses were not considered for analysis in the present study. The African respondents represented at least 20 ethnic groups hailing from 10 countries. As regards language, all except the participants from Rwanda and Burundi would have had their education in English starting from the secondary school level or earlier; and most of them would be at least bilingual.

Method of Analysis

The method of analysis used in this study was "thematic analysis". Put simply, "Thematic analysis is a method of identifying, analysing and reporting patterns

Table 6.1 Description of the data set

No.	Domains	Questions	N	E
1	Pregnancy and birthing rites	Describe the circumstances of your own conception and birth. What was said, the care given to your mother, and the expectations of the community? How is pregnancy related to the theme of creator God?	72	13
2	Naming rites	Describe the rituals by which you received your name. Who were you named after? What was said and done in the process of naming you? Was your name changed at any time after birth? Describe the person after whom you were named and indicate in what matter you are similar to him/her in terms of your personality, attitudes, looks and vocation. How is the naming process related to the theme of creator God?	75	15
3	Attitudes to sickness and ill health	What do you think and feel when you are not well? What do you feel is the cause of the problem? What does your community feel is the cause? What remedy(s) do you usually apply? What if the problem continues? Are the services of a diviner ever contemplated?	67	19
4	Formation and education	How were you formed and educated both informally and formally? Name as many as you can of the persons who were most influential in your own development. Indicate why they were important.	66	16
5	Initiation into adulthood rites	Describe how you were initiated into adulthood. How old were you, what were the rituals and rites that were performed? What was expected of you afterwards? How is the initiation process related to the theme of creator God and lineage ideology?	71	15
6	Marriage rites	Describe how you were married. How was your spouse selected, was there a person negotiating between your families, how was the bridewealth determined and paid, what were the various ceremonies and feasts that were held? (If not married, give the details of the ordinary marriage within your ethnic group.) How is marriage related to the themes of creator God and lineage ideology?	72	14
7	Mourning rites	Describe how you mourn and grieve at a funeral and the effect it has on the living. What is the meaning of mourning?	69	18
8	Inheritance ceremonies	How is the property, status and wife(s) [if patrilineal] of the deceased man inherited? When is this done? Is there a second funeral ceremony? What is the effect of inheritance ritual on an individual?	64	20
9	Elderhood rites	Describe the rites by which a person becomes a respected elder in your ethnic group. How is one selected, what is said and done? What are the instruments used, how is the feast organised, who is invited, what is expected of the elder afterwards? How is this domain related to the themes of creator God, lineage ideology, and witchcraft?	70	14
10	Funeral rites	Describe dying and death of a person in your ethnic group. What is said to explain the death? What are the major rituals? Is there a difference in the rituals and the rites if it is a man, woman or child? How is the grave dug? What is said at the gravesite? Is there a memorial feast at some later date? How is dying and death related to the themes of creator God, lineage ideology and witchcraft?	72	15

N number of participants, *E* number of ethnic groups represented in the sample

Table 6.2 The classification of values in action

	Core virtues	Character strengths
1	Wisdom and knowledge	Creativity (originality, ingenuity), curiosity (interest, novelty-seeking, openness to experience), open-mindedness (judgement, critical thinking), love of learning, perspective (wisdom)
2	Courage	Bravery (valour), persistence (perseverance, industriousness), integrity (authenticity, honesty), vitality (zest, enthusiasm, vigour, energy)
3	Humanity	Love, kindness (generosity, nurturance, care, compassion, altruistic love, "niceness"), social intelligence (emotional intelligence, personal intelligence)
4	Justice	Citizenship (social responsibility, loyalty, teamwork), fairness, leadership
5	Temperance	Forgiveness and mercy, humility (modesty), prudence, self-regulation (self-control)
6	Transcendence	Appreciation of beauty and excellence (awe, wonder, elevation), gratitude, hope (optimism, future-mindedness, future orientation), humour (playfulness), spirituality (religiousness, faith, purpose)

(themes) within data" (Braun and Clarke 2006: 79). Often, this approach goes beyond identifying and analysing to interpreting various aspects of the research topic (Boyatzis 1998). Thematic analysis is closely related to content analysis. Some scholars see thematic analysis as a technique of content analysis (Trochim and Donnelly 2006). While content analysis tends to be more systematic and mechanical (Eto and Kyngäs 2008; Hsieh and Shannon 2005), thematic analysis is more flexible and offers a possibility for theoretical openness and interpretation (Braun and Clarke 2006).

The present project took a hybrid approach of induction and deduction to thematic analysis (Fereday and Muir-Cochrane 2006). This approach is underpinned by the concept of "hermeneutic circle" that Gadamer (1979) borrowed from Heidegger. No interpreter (or researcher) comes to the text (data) with a mindset of "tabla rasa". The interpreter's pre-understandings become not just the starting point for interpretation but a condition for understanding. Therefore, while many theorists of qualitative research methods invite researchers to own up their "prejudices" in a reflexive process (Koppala and Suzuki 1999) in order to set them aside, in this project, the researchers embraced an explicit theoretical framework (positive psychology). However, after the data were interpreted, the possibility for the transformation or adjustment of the theoretical framework was also considered. This was in the spirit of what Gadamer (1979: 273) called "the fusion of horizons" but may be more correctly described as a "meeting of horizons".

In the present study, the theoretical framework of positive psychology acted as the coding template (Crabtree and Miller 1999). More precisely, the list of 6 core virtues and 24 character strengths (Peterson and Seligman 2004) together with their lexical equivalents (Table 6.2) were used. On the basis of this template, themes were initially identified within the data. The emerging patterns were then further used to

Fig. 6.1 Meeting of horizons in data analysis

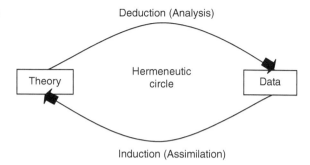

elaborate the codes. Having gone through this process, proposals were also made on possible contributions of African traditional religion to positive psychology. Thus, two distinct processes were at work (Fig. 6.1):

1. A deductive process of analysis: The data were analysed and interpreted using the template; this process was theory-driven.
2. An inductive process of assimilation: The possibility for the data to contribute to the reformulation of some aspects of the template was discussed; and this process was data-driven.

Procedure of Analysis

The deductive-inductive hybrid process as carried out in this study could be laid out in four stages as represented in Table 6.3. The table also explains briefly how the four steps were used in the present project. The present essay reports the outcome of these steps.

The analysis of the data itself consisted in applying the template of codes to the data set and picking up patterns in the data set. And this was carried out in the following steps:

The data set was initially read, domain after domain, with the coding template in mind. The purpose of this stage of reading was to get a general grasp of the tone of the data and to see if they have any correspondence to the coding template at all.

In the second round of reading, lexical expressions, descriptions of cultural institutions and conceptual equivalents in the data that had resemblance to the description of the character strengths were marked and assigned a code (see Table 6.4). For instance, here is a quote from the data set (Kirwen 2008: 193) reporting what an informant belonging to the Akamba ethnic group in Kenya had to say under the domain of elderhood rites (the italics shows phrases that were assigned codes by the researcher and verified by the secondary author):

> One becomes an elder after considering certain qualities. Mainly age, marital status, *discipline (CS8)*, *wisdom (CS5)*, wealth/success and experience which goes with the age. The community and also the existing elders choose an elder *(CS15)*. Before one becomes

Table 6.3 Tabular representation of the stages undertaken in the project

	Steps in thematic analysis[a]	Application of the steps in the research
Step 1	Identification of coding template	Description of character strengths within the theoretical framework of positive psychology
Step 2	Identification of the data set	Description of the anthropological data from the Maryknoll Institute, Nairobi
Step 3	Analysis of the data: identifying themes by applying the coding template to the data set	Identification of conceptual, lexical equivalents and patterns indicating the presence of character strengths in the data set, paying special attention to cultural institutions that sustain them
Step 4	Examining the identified themes: discussing their significance within context of the coding template	Further exploration of the conceptual and lexical equivalents by the use of other theoretical sources on ATR, in an attempt to understand them, and considering their possible contribution to the theoretical framework of positive psychology

[a]Adapted from Fereday and Muir-Cochrane (2006), who in turn adapt their steps from Boyatzis (1998) and Crabtree and Miller (1999)

an elder, he passes through certain rites of passage and rituals. At a certain point a ceremony is organized to welcome him to the council of elders. Afterwards he is given the *responsibility of being in charge of the community (CS13)*. Elderhood enhances the life process and directs the community *to the creator God (CS24)*, lineage and protects the lineage from witchcraft.

In this process of coding, particular attention was paid to cultural institutions, since it is one of the criteria used by positive psychology for the inclusion of any character strength in the "Manual of Sanities". The presence of cultural institutions shows that a given society places importance in the cultivation of that strength (Peterson and Seligman 2004; see also Biswas-Diener 2006).

At the third stage, a report was created for each of the CS picking up the marked phrases and sentences across the domains of the anthropological textual data. This formed the results section of the final report, which, in this essay, is significantly summarised. It was possible that one domain yielded data for more than one CS, and there were occasions when more than one domain yielded data for the same CS (see Table 6.4). The report was not just a listing of phrases but was in the form of meaningful sentences often integrating verbatim quotes. This implied certain degree of interpretation. However, care was taken to elucidate the expression of one participant with the help of the expressions from other participants within the same domain.

Results

For the sake of brevity, in this section, results are summarised in Table 6.4. Some typical statements are included below in the Discussion section to substantiate particular claims.

Table 6.4 Convergence of character strengths and African cultural religious domains

	D1, pregnancy and birthing rites	D2, naming rites	D3, attitudes to sickness and ill health	D4, formation and education	D5, initiation into adulthood rites	D6, marriage rites	D7, mourning rites	D8, inheritance ceremonies	D9, elderhood rites	D10, funeral rites
I. *Wisdom and knowledge*										
1 Creativity										
2 Curiosity										
3 Open-mindedness										
4 Love of learning				✔						
5 Perspective				✔	✔					
II. *Courage*										
6 Bravery					✔				✔	
7 Persistence									✔	
8 Integrity									✔	
9 Vitality										✔
III. *Humanity*										
10 Love						✔				
11 Kindness							✔			
12 Social intelligence									✔	
IV. *Justice*										
13 Citizenship				✔	✔	✔	✔		✔	
14 Fairness			✔					✔	✔	
15 Leadership										
V. *Temperance*										
16 Forgiveness and mercy										
17 Humility/modesty										
18 Prudence										
19 Self-regulation					✔				✔	
VI. *Transcendence*										
20 Appreciation of beauty	✔									
21 Gratitude	✔									
22 Hope										
23 Humour							✔			✔
24 Spirituality	✔	✔		✔	✔	✔	✔		✔	✔

Note: '✔' indicates that at least one participant used expressions that were similar to the description of the character strength in positive psychology

Eighteen out of the 24 character strengths were rated as showing some correspondence to the ten domains of the data set (Table 6.1). Out of these, eight CS showed correspondence to at least one of the domains, and others showed correspondence to more than one domain.

In general, two salient points emerged from the thematic analysis: (a) From the coding template, statements rated as corresponding to two character strengths (citizenship and spirituality) showed greater prevalence in the data set; (b) From among the anthropological domains, elderhood rites (D9) showed the greatest match to the character strengths.

Discussion

The absence of some of the character strengths in the present data set may not indicate their lack in the ATR. It is important to be aware that the data were not collected for the purpose of the study of the presence of character strengths. In addition, the data set used for the present study considered only the ten domains of the individual life cycle (Kirwen 2008). The Maryknoll Institute of African Studies (MIAS) has collected data for 25 domains drawn from a further three cycles, namely, family and interpersonal relationships cycle, community and communal activities cycle and religious rituals cycle.

It is possible that the greater prevalence of spirituality (CS24) in the data set has been a result of a bias in the questions presented to the participants. Out of the ten questions (see Table 6.1), six had a precise mention of "the creator God". Nonetheless, since the data used for the present analysis were collected for a very generic purpose, the consistent prevalence of spirituality in the data set could also reflect the world view of the general population. Does the high prevalence of citizenship say something significant about the world view of ATR? Citizenship includes social responsibility and loyalty and represents general commitment to common good. Is this CS really strong in the African religion and culture? And what is the significance of elderhood in relation to the CS of positive psychology? In what follows, we answer these questions and others, generating a dialogue between the present data set and other scholarly works in an attempt to validate our interpretation.

It Takes a Village: The Context and Purpose of Wisdom and Knowledge

The character strengths of wisdom and knowledge cannot be understood in the African context apart from the community. It is in the framework of the community that an individual acquires wisdom and knowledge. No wonder Hillary Clinton chose a phrase from a West African proverb for the title of her book on welfare of children and family: "It takes a village to educate a child" (Clinton 1996). As it has emerged from the data set, the process of acquiring knowledge is informal and done in the context of the family, though there are also formal moments like the preparation for initiation (Mosha 2000). The purpose of knowledge is for the well-being of the community within which individuals find their own well-being. One Tigrinya-speaking participant (from Eritrea) offers a succinct summary of this core virtue under the domain of "formation and education" (Kirwen 2008: 76): "Although the contribution of the larger community cannot be ignored, my parents played a critical role both in my informal and formal education. At an early age they taught me to fear God. They instilled in me the values of honesty and truthfulness, respect for elders, and love for learning and seeking wisdom".

One of the points of divergence between the empirical findings in positive psychology and the anthropological data about ATR is the correlation between age and wisdom. In some adult samples, relationship between chronological age and wisdom-related knowledge was non-significant (Pasupathi et al. 2001). Many respondents in the present study consistently related wisdom to mature age and elderhood. For instance, a Luo informant from Kenya states, "In my tribe, one becomes a respected elder because of his sense of responsibility, his age and wisdom" (Kirwen 2008: 192). However, no mention of chronological age was made. On the other hand, in his attempt to develop an "African sagacity", some of the "sages" that the African scholar Oruka interviewed were in their forties (Oruka 1990). Moreover, according to Magesa (1998), any initiated person is potentially an elder. Therefore, we can conceptually assume that also in the African world view, wisdom is related to maturity and elderhood and not necessarily to chronological age.

Abundant Life: African "Vitalogy" as the Basis for Courage and Integrity

The character strengths that are grouped under the core virtue of courage feature strongly in the ATR. The initiation ritual is accompanied by an element of physical pain: whether it is the most common ritual of circumcision or the extraction of teeth (among the Luos and other Nilotic peoples) or tattooing (among the Teso) or making incisions on the head (among the Nuba). The young initiates are expected to be "bold" (Kirwen 2008: 103), to pass through this immediate pain, so that they would be able to enjoy the privileges of being an adult in their community. The descriptions of the elderhood rites in ATR allude to the understanding that the elder is an exemplar of bravery. While physical valour would be the pride of younger warriors, bravery of the elder would be seen in his ability "to settle disputes or represent the clan in matters that required negotiation among [other] elders" (Kirwen 2008: 193). In the ATR, formation and education consists not only in learning knowledge and skills but also in acquiring values, especially of "honesty and truthfulness" (Kirwen 2008: 76). In the selection of elders, besides wisdom, as reported above, integrity is another important criterion. There is a consistent voice among the respondents about "the moral uprightness" of the elder: "The elder was expected to live an exemplary life – no arguments or quarrelling, not greedy, not corrupt, above lies and having an enhanced ability of keeping his wife and children under control" (Agikuyu informant from Kenya, in Kirwen 2008: 195).

The character strength of vitality deserves a special mention. In positive psychology, vitality consists in "…living life as an adventure; feeling alive and activated" (Peterson 2006: 32). In the present data, it is the African attitude towards death, expressed in the funeral rites, which brings out their attitude towards life. While "the death of elder is celebrated as the culmination of a life fully lived" (Kirwen 2008: 224), and that of a warrior is marked by "dancing and eating to send [him] off", suicide is "handled very seriously with plenty of cleansing and destruction of the deceased's home" (Kirwen 2008: 228). Placide Tempels (1959) in his groundbreaking work, *La Philosophie Bantoue*, had introduced the concept of "the vital force" (see also Taylor 1963: 51). While Magesa (1998) develops an African norm of morality based on the principle of "abundant life", Nkemnkia (1999) proposes "vitalogy" as the central concept in African philosophy. In this light, the inclusion by positive psychology of vitality as a character strength under the core virtue of courage seems not appropriate. Perhaps "vitality" could be a generic construct, which in turn could be the basis for courage and integrity.

There Is One More Place: African Expressions of Humanity

Taylor (1963: 188) concludes his book, with a succinct assertion about "the primal vision" of the African world view: "Africans believe that presence is the debt they owe to one another". "Presence" could be suggested as a one-word summary for the character strengths listed in VIA under the virtue of "humanity": love, kindness and social intelligence. In the African traditional religions, mourning rituals powerfully express kindness and compassion as understood by positive psychology. It is in this domain that a large manifestation of agreement was noticed among the participants. These expressions of kindness and compassion range from being "nice" to the dead to showing solidarity by being "present" with the living. These twin aspects are affirmed by many respondents: "Talking nicely about the departed is a way of mourning" (Kirwen 2008: 151), and "mourning is a sign of great loss and companionship to the bereaved family" (p. 152). It is important to note that during the period of mourning, the neighbours and relatives physically spend most of the time together with the bereaved, as a Dinka (Sudan) respondent voices: "[mourning] involves wailing and living at the home of the deceased for four days" (p. 153).

African society is generally inclusive and welcoming. Whether it is in the bus, or at the table, there is always one more place for anyone. In African sagacity, happiness itself is defined as being open to all people (Oruka 1990: 112). A concrete expression of this openness and presence is hospitality (Healey 1981). Strangely, hospitality has not received much attention within positive psychology. This could be another meaningful contrition from ATR to character strengths.

The African sense of inclusiveness is also seen in the way people express their opinion. This can be considered the core of African social intelligence. During meetings, points are not debated as in a Western parliament, but everyone adds data to the common search for truth and meaning (Donders 1985). This theme of "consensus-seeking" could be a valuable contribution from ATR to the character strength of social intelligence in PP. The African elder then is expected to be endowed with a great degree of social intelligence. He plays a vital role in consensus building. The elder "is selected on the merit of being straightforward" (a Tutsi respondent, Kirwen 2008: 196); similarly, he is also expected to be "mature, respectable, obedient, kind and loving" (An Agikuyu participant, Kirwen 2008: 197).

I Am Because We Are: African Citizenship, Leadership and Justice

As it has been stated previously, the African identity and virtue – being and functioning – emanate from the context of the community. Mbiti (1969: 108–109) affirms, "Whatever happens to the individual happens to the whole group, and whatever happens to the whole group happens to the individual. The individual can only say: 'I am, because we are; and since we are, therefore I am'. This is a cardinal point in understanding the African view of man". This view is rephrased by a Nigerian scholar, "I am because I belong" (Metuh 1985: 99), or as Taylor (1963: 85) put it, "I am because I participate". In this sense, the character strengths that are grouped by PP under the core virtue of justice, together with those under the virtue of humanity (love, kindness and social intelligence), form the core of the African world view. In the data analysis, in addition to bravery, initiation rites were seen to be related also to the character strength of responsibility or citizenship: "I was initiated to adulthood through circumcision at fourteen years. I was secluded for one month for training to be responsible..." (an Agikuyu participant, Kirwen 2008: 103).

This is also supported by Mbiti's claim (1969: 121) that through the initiation rites, "they enter into a state of responsibility: they inherit new rights, and new obligations are expected of them by society". On the other hand, leadership is attributed to the role of the elders. The observation of Magesa (1998: 71) regarding African leadership is relevant to explain this character strength: Leadership is concerned with enhancing life; it is communal – always bringing people together; it is caring for the whole of life – spiritual and secular.

Also, African marriage is communal (Kirwen 2008: 126, 133). In the parlance of our coding template, we can say that marriage represents a general commitment to the common good: "Marriage is seen as a way of bringing a man and woman together to give the community children who will carry on the name of the family" (a Teso participant from Kenya, Kirwen 2008: 126). The theme of moral reasoning as an aspect of fairness emerges very explicitly in the African attitude to sickness and ill health. Several responses in the data set show that someone who is ill would perceive a moral implication in their condition, particularly examining their own moral role in the sickness, even if infection of some kind could be the immediate cause: "I have neglected my social responsibilities" (p. 57); or "sickness is a curse which one receives after disowning certain rules and rites of the society"

(p. 58); "I wonder whether I have wronged someone" (p. 59); "it is due to some mistake that I did or as a result of sin" (p. 60). "The community will want to find out what mistake I have done and there are also feelings that someone is behind my sickness" (a Dinka from the Sudan, p. 65). Against this background, "the remedy is to take medicine, that is Western or herbal. If the problem persists, I may seek the services of the diviner" (an Akamba participant from Kenya, p. 62). The role of the diviner is sought, not only to find the real cause of the sickness but also to mediate reconciliation between conflicting parties in such a way that the social order that was disrupted by the transgression may now be restored.

Maintaining Communion: Regulation and Reconciliation

Self-regulation as a character strength of temperance, according to positive psychology, is also referred to as self-control or self-discipline. Self-regulation is marked by a readiness for delayed gratification. In ATR, the preparation towards the initiation ceremony could be seen as a cultural institution to instil the need for self-discipline. The young initiates are expected to endure immediate pain, so that they would be able to enjoy the privileges of being an adult in their community. Discipline is also considered as one of the salient virtues of an elder. An Akamba respondent from Kenya affirms, "A person becomes an elder first by virtue of his age and discipline" (Kirwen 2008: 191, see also p. 193).

Though the data set used for the present analysis, perhaps prejudiced by the anthropological domains and their related questions, did not show any direct allusion to the theme of forgiveness, many other anthropological discussions on ATR do make reference to this theme. Reconciliation is seen as behavioural and attitudinal changes that are "intended to re-establish harmony and equilibrium of life" (Magesa 1998: 208). This process, even if often it could be only between individuals, is facilitated by the community through rituals and external signs. For instance, what is achieved in gesture and word through the performance of a ritual called *kutasa* among the Taita people of Kenya has to be matched by the person's inner state of freedom from anger (Harris 1978: 28). Similar rituals are reported among the Nyakusa of Tanzania (Wilson 1971). Among the Chagga people of Tanzania, the exchange of the leaves of Isale – dracaena trees – as a sign of reconciliation is also well known (Healey and Sybertz 1996: 316–317). Other character strengths listed under the virtue of temperance need further exploration.

Being Notoriously Religious: A Spirituality of Life

"Africans are notoriously religious, and each people has its own religious system with a set of beliefs and practices....African peoples do not know how to exist without religion" (Mbiti 1969: 1–2). In the opinion of a non-African scholar,

Parrinder (1954/1974: 9), "What are the forces behind these surging peoples of Africa? One of the greatest forces has ever been the power of religion. 'This incurably religious people' was a phrase often on the lips of many old [colonial] administrators". A similar finding emerged also in this study. From birth rites to funeral rites, almost all character strengths were seen to be related to the spiritual realm. For instance, the respondents are almost unanimous in their claim that the African societies see pregnancy and birth as "a blessing from God". An Akamba participant affirms, "Pregnancy is the start of life and it is sacred and the process is God given" (Kirwen 2008: 14). In naming rites, there are expressions of the individuals' link with reality beyond themselves – in this case, the link to the generation's past. One Aembu respondent offers a typical summary: "There is a comprehensive scheme of naming children after maternal and paternal relatives – dead or alive. Names give social identity to a child. Naming is a rite of incorporation in which the sacred is pivotal" (p. 37). Formation and education is associated with fear of God. One respondent recalls that his or her parents played a critical role in their "informal and formal education. At an early age they taught me to fear God..." (p. 76). Many of the initiation ceremonies described by participants relate to shedding of blood of the initiate. "The shedding of the blood [was] to unite me to the lineage" (p. 101). This, together with animal sacrifice, can be considered as cultural institutions that express transcendence. Again, in the understanding of marriage in Africa, and the rituals that accompany it, there is an underlying conviction that there is a transcendental dimension of marriage, and that marriage is an event that fits into the larger scheme of life. "God is seen as the one who arranges marriage" (p. 123), and "marriage is a gift (or a blessing) from God where life is expressed" (p. 125). The sacredness (p. 134) of marriage is particularly expressed in the sacrifice and libation performed (p. 124), which signify that marriage is a bridge between God, the ancestors, the couple and community at large and the yet unborn (pp. 131–132). Expressions of transcendence are seen in the domain of mourning rites, not in a direct relationship with God but "mourning symbolizes companionship with the dead whose spirit is still believed to be around" (p. 150). And some "people believe that there is no death as such but [only] passing over to the spirit world" (p. 153). These expressions allude to the unswerving faith of the African peoples in a reality beyond the here and now. In the domain of elderhood rites, on the one hand, during his lifetime, the elder is considered a representative of God (p. 194); that is why the installation of the elder involves offering of sacrifice and libation (p. 195). On the other hand, after his death, he becomes an ancestor who continues to mediate between God and the people (p. 193). African spirituality is also demonstrated in the peoples' attitude towards death. Even if there is initial mourning, there is an acceptance of the event: "God is the giver and taker of life". This concept is repeated in almost every page of the participants' description of funeral rites (pp. 223–235). This consolation comes from the fact that dead people, if they lived a virtuous life, are considered ancestors (p. 226). Sacrifice and libation give the possibility for the living to commune with them (p. 230).

Besides the CS of spirituality, the other character strengths of transcendence are also prevalent. Rituals found in the African mourning rites seem to allude powerfully to the African expressions of hope. Several respondents representing various ethnic groups mention "shaving of head" or "cutting of hair" as one of the rituals accompanying mourning (Abaluyia, p. 151; Baganda, p. 152; Kipsigis, p. 152; Luo, p. 153; Tigrinya, p. 153, just to site the most salient). This ritual could be seen as a "form of self-punishing behaviour" (as noted by a Tigrinya respondent, p. 153) or as "a sign of innocence, i.e., you have nothing to do with the death" – that is, you have not caused the death (as claimed by an Abaluyia respondent, p. 151), or "as a sign of helplessness and weakness" together with smearing of ashes (as noted by a Luo respondent, p. 156). However, this ritual could also be interpreted as a sign of hope that the hair that is now cut will eventually grow again and life will go on. This is supported by scholars like Magesa (1998: 150): Hair is a symbol of life because of its continued growth. "When the hair grows back – and this is what the ritual also says – the life of family and clan, now aided by the new life force of the deceased relative, must continue and thrive".

In the study by Biswas-Diener (2006: 300, 302), all of the Maasai participants ($N = 123$) endorsed "appreciation of beauty" as an existing virtue in their society, but they also pointed out that there is no cultural institution among them related to appreciation of beauty. In the present data, appreciation of beauty featured only in the domain of pregnancy. Other aspects of transcendence, like optimism, hope and humour, which did not emerge strongly in the present study, may be found in ATR, but this needs further study. For instance, "hakuna matata", a Swahili phrase popularised by the Disney film *Lion King*, means "there is no problem". This is not just a jargon but an attitude in Africa. African greetings consistently and explicitly make use of positive phrases (Healey 1981: 156). In brief, most scholars claim that spirituality permeates almost every aspect of African life (Magesa 1998).

The African Elder: A Paragon of Character Strengths

Another interesting finding that emerged from this qualitative research was the figure of the African elder and its association to character strengths. The domain of the elderhood rites shows association with at least eight of the character strengths, stretching across all core virtues (Table 6.4). The elder is expected to be endowed with wisdom. This wisdom is an outcome of experience and reflection. The elder is also an exemplar of courage, especially in "speaking up for what is right" (Peterson 2006: 32). The elder is also known for his integrity: upright, exemplary and refined in his dealing with others. This moral standard provides him the authority to advice others – a trait of social intelligence. In a possible leadership role, the elder is able to influence the community in decision making and is able to inspire others. In short, he is the paragon of character strengths (see Peterson and Seligman 2004: 24). As Magesa (1998) states, the African elder is not necessarily a leader in a social or political sense. Since in the African world view religion is not separate from society, the elder could also play the role of a diviner, a priest or a medium. In the world of the living, he mediates between God and the community. And in death, he joins the living dead and becomes immortal. He lives in the memory of the community as an ancestor.

Concluding Remarks

Norenzayan and Heine (2005: 766) propose cross-fertilisation between anthropology and psychology in the study of "psychological universals". They acknowledge the importance of strategies that will facilitate cross-cultural discourse while respecting the "idiosyncrasies of psychological research". This research project was meant to be a modest contribution to the ongoing discussion on the ubiquity of core virtues and character strengths of positive psychology drawing evidence from cross-cultural data. Insofar as the project reinterprets the beliefs, codes and cults of ATR in the contemporary parlance of psychology, this study also makes a contribution to the discourse of ATR.

The most meaningful way of studying a traditional religion was to use anthropological data, even if that data came from students who were educated in the Western system. This background of the participants who contributed to the data needs to be considered in the light of how ATR works. As Magesa (1998) explains, African religious perspectives persist even among the African adherents of Christianity because ATR is not a structured religion but a spirituality and a world view (see also Shorter 1973). It is spirituality insofar as ATR influences people's relation to the Higher Power, and it is a world view inasmuch as it governs the way the African people interpret the reality around them.

In the analysis of the sampled anthropological data, it was also more convenient to use a qualitative method of analysis, as it is increasingly being used in cross-cultural studies in positive psychology (Delle Fave and Bassi 2009b). Ong and van Dulmen (2007) consider the possibility of integrating quantitative and qualitative approaches in positive psychology. Besides, as Robbins (2008: 96) contends, "Eudaimonic happiness cannot be purely value-free, nor can it be completely studied without using both nomothetic and idiographic (i.e., quantitative and qualitative) methods in addressing problems of value…".

In qualitative research the influence of researcher's subjectivity is inevitable, particularly given the fact that the primary researcher has spent 16 years in East Africa. The focus in this work was on how this subjectivity could be meaningfully used in analysis (Sciarra 1998). The role of the secondary researcher, who has interests in psychology of religion and positive psychology, has contributed to improve the reliability of the findings. Several other aspects that enhance the "validity" of qualitative research (Merrick 1998; Yardley 2008) have been taken into account in this project. The researchers have been transparent about the method of qualitative thematic analysis that was employed in this project. The discussion section of the project has employed a type of triangulation, by way of a modest literature review of other scholarship. In any case, since both the coding templates and the data set came from previous scholarship, at least the stages of data collection and framing of codes have not been contaminated by the research questions or the subjective influence of the researchers.

Peterson (2006) agrees that the Values in Action (VIA) is still a work in progress. Therefore, of particular importance would be further study of specific concepts that have emerged in the present study: For instance, could hospitality and "presence" be character strengths within the core virtue of humanity? Again, some character strengths that have direct moral implications like integrity and fairness are found to be classified in the VIA under core virtues of courage and justice respectively. During this study, it was found that, on the one hand, the core virtue of "courage" does not best represent the character strengths that are listed therein; on the other hand, integrity might need a shift to the core virtue of justice. We suggest this needs further examination.

The present work studied only the first volume of data, collected by MIAS, Nairobi, pertaining to individual life cycle, covering ten anthropological domains. MIAS has data in three other volumes (Kirwen 2005) on family and interpersonal relationship cycle, community and communal activities cycle and religious ritual cycle, covering 35 domains in all. It would be fruitful to expand this present work to analyse data from all domains.

In general, this qualitative study has shown that more cross-cultural studies are needed on the VIA so that the list might be enhanced in the light of their findings, and thus provide a universal and culturally fair perspective on good and engaged life.

Acknowledgements A previous version of this chapter was presented at the 5th European Conference on Positive Psychology, June 23–26, 2010, Copenhagen, Denmark. The authors are grateful to Dr. Adrian Coyle (Surrey University, UK) and Dr. Michael Kirwen (Maryknoll Institute of African Studies, Nairobi) for their assistance in the dissertation project of the first author, which this essay reports.

References

Beugré, C., & Offodile, O. (2001). Managing for organizational effectiveness in sub-Saharan Africa: A culture-fit model. *International Journal of Human Resource Management, 12*, 535–550.

Biswas-Diener, R. (2006). From the equator to the north pole: A study of character strengths. *Journal of Happiness Studies, 7*, 293–310.

Boyatzis, R. E. (1998). *Transforming qualitative information: Thematic analysis and code development*. London: Sage.

Braun, V., & Clarke, V. (2006). Using thematic analysis in psychology. *Qualitative Research in Psychology, 3*, 77–101.

Chu, K., & Diener, E. (2009). Religion as a source of variation in the experience of positive and negative emotions. *The Journal of Positive Psychology, 4*, 447–460.

Clinton, H. R. (1996). *It takes a village*. New York: Simon & Schuster.

Coetzee, S., & Viviers, R. (2007). An overview of research on positive psychology in South Africa. *South African Journal of Psychology, 37*, 470–490.

Cox, J. L. (2007). *From primitive to indigenous: The academic study of indigenous religions*. Surrey: Ashgate Publishing.

Crabtree, B., & Miller, W. (1999). A template approach to text analysis: Developing and using codebooks. In B. Crabtree & W. Miller (Eds.), *Doing qualitative research* (pp. 163–177). Thousand Oaks: Sage Publications.

Dahlsgaard, K., Peterson, C., & Seligman, M. E. P. (2005). Shared virtue: The convergence of valued human strengths across culture and history. *Review of General Psychology, 9*, 203–213.

Delle Fave, A., & Bassi, M. (2009a). The contribution of diversity to happiness research. *The Journal of Positive Psychology, 4*, 205–207.

Delle Fave, A., & Bassi, M. (2009b). Sharing optimal experiences and promoting good community life in a multicultural society. *The Journal of Positive Psychology, 4*, 280–289.

Donders, J. G. (1985). *Non-bourgeois theology: An African experience of Jesus*. Maryknoll: Orbis Books.

Durkheim, E. (1915). *Elementary forms of the religious life: A study of religious sociology*. London: Allen & Unwin.

Eloff, I. (2008). Editorial–positive psychology: Celebrating strength and well-being in the cradle of humankind. *Journal of Psychology in Africa, 18*, 5–8.

Eto, S., & Kyngäs, H. (2008). The qualitative content analysis process. *Journal of Advanced Nursing, 62*, 107–115.

Evans-Pritchard, E. E. (1965). *Theories of primitive religion*. Oxford: Clarendon.

Fereday, J., & Muir-Cochrane, E. (2006). Demonstrating rigor using thematic analysis: A hybrid approach of inductive and deductive coding and theme development. *International Journal of Qualitative Methods, 5*, 1–11.

Gadamer, H. (1979). *Truth and method*. London: Sheed & Ward.

Haidt, J. (2003). Elevation and the positive psychology of morality. In C. L. M. Keyes & J. Haidt (Eds.), *Flourishing: Positive psychology and the life well-lived* (pp. 275–289). Washington, DC: American Psychological Association.

Harris, G. G. (1978). *Casting out anger: Religion among the Taita of Kenya*. Cambridge: Cambridge University Press.

Healey, J. G. (1981). *The fifth gospel: In search of black Christian values*. London: SCM Press.

Healey, J. G., & Sybertz, D. F. (1996). *Towards an African narrative theology*. Nairobi: Pauline Publications.

Hsieh, H., & Shannon, S. (2005). Three approaches to qualitative content analysis. *Qualitative Health Research, 15*, 1277–1288.

Idowu, E. B. (1973). *African traditional religion: A definition*. London: SCM Press.

Joseph, S., Linley, P. A., & Matlby, J. (2006). Positive psychology, religion, and spirituality. *Mental Health, Religion and Culture, 9*, 209–212.

Kirwen, M. C. (Ed.). (2005). *African cultural knowledge: Themes and embedded beliefs*. Nairobi: Maryknoll Institute of African Studies.

Kirwen, M. C. (Ed.). (2008). *African cultural domains: Life cycle of an individual*. Nairobi: Maryknoll Institute of African Studies.

Koppala, M., & Suzuki, L. A. (1999). *Using Qualitative Methods in Psychology*. London: Sage.

Lowie, R. H. (1924). *Primitive Religion*. New York: Boni & Liveright.

Magesa, L. (1998). *African religion: The moral traditions of abundant life*. Nairobi: Paulines Publications.

Maltby, L., & Hill, P. (2008). 'So firm a foundation': What the comparative study of religion offers positive psychology. *Research in the Social Scientific Study of Religion, 19*, 117–142.

Mazrui, A. A. (1986). *The Africans: A triple heritage*. London: BBC Publications.

Mbiti, J. S. (1969). *African religions and philosophy*. Nairobi: East African Educational Publishers.

McCullough, M., & Snyder, C. (2000). Classical source of human strength: Revisiting an old home and building a new one. *Journal of Social and Clinical Psychology, 19*, 1–10.

Merrick, E. (1998). An exploration of quality in qualitative research: Are "reliability" and "validity" relevant? In M. Kopala & L. A. Suzuki (Eds.). *Using qualitative methods in Psychology* (pp. 25–36). London: Sage Publications.

Metuh, E. I. (1985). *African religions in western conceptual schemes: The problem of interpretation*. Ibadan: Pastoral Institute.

Mosha, R. S. (2000). *The heartbeat of indigenous Africa: A study of Chagga educational system*. London: Routledge.

Nansook, P., Peterson, C., & Seligman, M. E. P. (2006). Character strengths in fifty-four nations and the fifty US states. *The Journal of Positive Psychology, 1*, 118–129.

Nkemnkia, M. N. (1999). *African Vitalogy: A step forward in African thinking*. Nairobi: Paulines.

Norenzayan, A., & Heine, S. (2005). Psychological universals: What are they and how can we know? *Psychological Bulletin, 131*, 763–784.

Ong, A. D., & van Dulman, M. H. M. (2007). *Oxford handbook of methods in positive psychology*. New York: Oxford University Press.

Oruka, H. O. (1990). *Sage philosophy: Indigenous thinkers and modern debate on African philosophy*. Leiden: E.J. Brill.

P'Bitek, O. (1970). *African religions in western scholarship*. Kampala: East African Literature Bureau.

Park, N., & Peterson, C. (2007). Methodological issues in positive psychology and the assessment of character strengths. In A. D. Ong & M. H. M. van Dulman (Eds.), *Oxford handbook of methods in positive psychology* (pp. 292–305). New York: Oxford University Press.

Parrinder, G. I. (1954/1974). *African traditional religion* (3rd ed.). London: Sheldon Press.

Pasupathi, M., Staudinger, U., & Baltes, P. (2001). Seeds of wisdom: Adolescents' knowledge and judgment about difficult life problems. *Developmental Psychology, 37*, 351–361.

Peterson, C. (2006). Values in action (VIA): Classification of strengths. In M. Csikszentmihalyi & I. S. Csikszentmihalyi (Eds.), *A life worth living: Contributions to positive psychology* (pp. 29–48). Oxford: Oxford University Press.

Peterson, C., & Seligman, M. E. P. (2004). *Character strengths and virtues: A handbook and classification*. Oxford: Oxford University Press.

Robbins, B. (2008). What is the good life? Positive psychology and the renaissance of humanistic psychology. *Humanistic Psychologist, 36*, 96–112.

Sciarra, D. (1998). The role of the qualitative researcher. In M. Kopala & L. A. Suzuki (Eds.), *Using qualitative methods in Psychology* (pp. 38–48). London: Sage Publications.

Selvam, S. G. (2008). A capabilities approach to youth rights in East Africa. *The International Journal of Human Rights, 12*, 205–214.

Shillington, K. (2005). *Encyclopedia of Africa history*. San Francisco: CRC Press.

Shorter, A. (1973). *African culture and the Christian church*. London: Geoffrey Chapman.

Shorter, A. (1975). Problems and possibilities for the Church's dialogue with African traditional religion. In A. Shorter (Ed.), *Dialogue with the African traditional religions*. Kampala: Gaba Publications.

Snyder, C. R., & Lopez, S. J. (2007). *Positive psychology: The scientific and practical explorations of human strength*. Thousand Oaks: SAGE Publications.

Sundararajan, L. (2005). Happiness donut: A Confucian critique of positive psychology. *Journal of Theoretical and Philosophical Psychology, 25*, 35–60.

Taylor, J. V. (1963). *The primal vision: Christian presence amid African religion*. London: SCM Press.

Tempels, P. (1959). *Bantu Philosophy*. Paris: Présence Africaine.

Trochim, W., & Donnelly, J. P. (2006). *The research methods knowledge base*. Mason: Atomic Dog.

Tylor, E. B. (1871/1958). *Primitive culture*. New York: Harper & Row.

Vitz, P. (2005). Psychology in recovery. *First Things: A Monthly Journal of Religion & Public Life, 151*, 17–21.

Watts, F., Dutton, K., & Gulliford, L. (2006). Human spiritual qualities: Integrating psychology and religion. *Mental Health, Religion and Culture, 9*, 277–289.

Wilson, M. (1971). *Religion and the transformation of society: A study in social change in Africa*. Cambridge: Cambridge University Press.

Yardley, L. (2008). Demonstrating validity in qualitative psychology. In J. A. Smith (Ed.), *Qualitative psychology: A practical guide to research methods* (2nd ed., pp. 235–251). London: Sage.

Zagano, P., & Gillespie, C. K. (2006). Ignatian spirituality and positive psychology. *The Way, 45*, 41–48.

Chapter 7
Culture, Environmental Psychology, and Well-Being: An Emergent Theoretical Framework

Nicola Rainisio and Paolo Inghilleri

Natures, Cultures, and Well-Being

Nature is one of the most complex and polysemic concepts for human imagination, and any attribution of meaning is therefore subject to considerable variability.

As stated by Redclift (2003), "nature is now one of the most contested domains of the human choice, subject to interpretation and invoked as moral justification, in a world of rival epistemologies (…)" (p. 177). In particular, there are two main sources of this variability: time and place.

Some scholars in environmental history underlined an evolution of the concept of nature in the course of time inside the Western culture.

Nash (1967), writing about *wilderness*, suggested that it was historically associated with negative meanings coming from the Judaic-Christian religious tradition, which were later successfully transformed to take on a positive representation when the industrial revolution was completed and the US culture created a new "myth of origin."

Merchant (2003) also stressed that the Western world is trying to *reconstruct the Eden*, by subscribing to a new paradigm based on a "return to nature" after the original sin of industrialization.

According to Sieferle (2003, p. 22), we can even "observe nature changing political sides, from political right to political left" in the nineteenth century, when the spread of evolutionary theory was linked to a possibility of social progress for workers and the primacy of science and technology over religion had been claimed.

Ehlers (2003) too agrees that the way of considering nature during the late nineteenth century has changed: the city became the only space apt to symbolize the profane, while the cultivated nature acquired its original structural order and wild

N. Rainisio (✉) • P. Inghilleri
Department of Cultural Heritage and Environment,
Università degli Studi di Milano, Milan, Italy
e-mail: nicola.rainisio@unimi.it; paolo.inghilleri@unimi.it

H.H. Knoop and A. Delle Fave (eds.), *Well-Being and Cultures: Perspectives from Positive Psychology*, Cross-Cultural Advancements in Positive Psychology 3, DOI 10.1007/978-94-007-4611-4_7, © Springer Science+Business Media Dordrecht 2013

nature turned into a *sacred* place, a place for mental and physical recreation and conservation values.

Moreover, he states that the ancient urban-wilderness dynamic has been completely reversed by the actual representation of nature. It is the contemporary city, *the concrete jungle*, that is, as wild as a mysterious forest of symbols, while the ecological ideals guide a threatened nature to new forms of absolute protection.

Besides these diachronic changes, the concept of nature is also subject to synchronic ones: it varies according to local sociocultural contexts.

This process occurs in two ways: inside the same cultural system and in the comparison between different cultures.

The main example of the first is the environmentalist paradigm, born as a subculture in the 1960s, and today affirmed as a mainstream narrative in our postmodern society.

A comparison between cultures has also underlined significant differences. Hong-key Yoon (2003, p. 139) affirmed:

> Therefore dichotomy of humanity (culture) and nature (the environment) is an important characteristic of the Western ideas. In contrast, Eastern ideas are based on monism and assume that people and the environment are two different expressions of the same entity.

Moreover, Western culture has supported a vision based on a determinist relationship between nature and culture, although changing the overriding factor according to the theories of reference, while the Eastern one has preferred a bidirectionality and mutual interdependence.

As a result, every culture has developed a peculiar *geomentality*, which can be traced by analyzing the human organization of nature, for example, in the history of agriculture and of gardening.

By avoiding any *radical constructivism* (Von Glasersfeld 1984) that involves the risk of underestimating the degradation of nature as a "real" physical entity, it is then possible to affirm that nature is an *artifact* (Vygotskij 1934/1962; Inghilleri 1999) that contains and conveys cultural information.

This symbolic nature is a *meme* (Dawkins 1976) that is subject to change over time and place.

Due to these features, it is also possible to identify universal representations, images, and values of nature shared worldwide.

The main among these is related to the positive effects of nature on subjective and social well-being, a widespread belief deeply rooted in popular learning.

Minteer and Manning (1999), in a study of natural values, mentioned the quality of life as one of the most important shared concerns regarding nature, as the large majority of environmental psychologists agree with the existence of a "natural effect" on physiology, attention, and cognitive abilities.

The same effects have been reported in Western culture through literature (with the Romantic Movement) by poets, such as William Blake, and philosophers, such as Immanuel Kant, starting from the eighteenth century. On the other hand, these effects were known since ancient times in Eastern cultural traditions.

For example, the Chinese fashionable practice called Feng Shui is based on a metaphorical comparison between body and landscape, in which the free flow of terrestrial energy is supposedly able to enhance mental and physical health.

It is noteworthy that almost all human cultures recognize trees and plants as primary sources for therapeutic purposes, also attributing several special healing powers to specific natural places and making them objects of devotion and ritual pilgrimages.

In this regard, Gesler has coined the term therapeutic landscapes to define those places where "the natural and built physical environments, social conditions and human perception interact to create an atmosphere that is conductive to healing" (1996, p. 96).

Cross-Cultural Research on Nature

The relationship between human beings and the environment, and its role in the process of community well-being, varies according to the cultural affiliations. Cultures are supposed to be a framework for different representations of nature.

The way people perceive and use the environment is, in large part, encouraged or limited by social norms and collective representations they have borrowed within their cultural context.

Kluckhohn and Strodtbeck (1961) in their well-known values orientation theory proposed that all human beings must answer to a limited number of universal problems. One of them is the relationship with the natural environment. Their taxonomy suggested that cultures can differ in the tendency to conceptualize that relationship in terms of subjugation, harmony, or mastery.

A similar typology is still used in contemporary research: Kellert (1995) proposes ten basic attitudes to compare the Japanese and the American culture. The results suggested some important differences in the cultural approach: Japanese people seemed to prefer managed settings where they could apply their shared attitudes to control and master the wildlife, whereas Americans showed a wider inclination toward ecological and moralistic values.

The influence of culture on the perception of the natural environment is particularly evident when members of different cultures use the same natural setting. As in the case of migration, the underlying *hidden dimension* of rules that regulate the space become clear in fostering the adoption of either new forms of relationship with the land or, alternatively, of attitudes in opposition to the dominant ones. Buijs and colleagues (2009) identify substantial cultural differences in place preferences.

Analyzing a sample with native Dutch and Muslim immigrants, the first group showed a preference for wild landscapes, while the second one expressed a clear preference for managed nature. The authors explained this result with the existence of cultural differences in the images of nature inside the Islamic and the Christian cultures, whereas "many immigrants supported the functional image of nature, with its focus on utilitarian values and intensive management. This may be related to the divine task in Islam for humans to manage nature and to bring wild areas into culture" (p. 9). It is noteworthy that the imaginary of immigrants of second generation, born or educated in the new country, is closer to the autochthonous perception, indicating that there has been a process of internalization of significant parts of a new cultural paradigm (e.g., Berry 1980).

Research on leisure highlighted ethnical particularities in the participation and behaviors of minorities in natural areas. Two recent reviews (Byrne and Wolch 2009; Floyd et al. 2008) stated significant differences within the American subgroups (Hispanics, Afro-American, Asiatic, Anglos) regarding the activities, the group dynamics, and the reasons underlying the visits to parks and green areas.

For example, Kaplan and Talbot (1988) observed that African Americans preferred more structured settings than Whites, whereas the Latinos (Chavez 2001) tended to choose environments able to promote a higher level of socialization and interaction with the others.

These results have been explained by several theoretical frameworks, the first of which proposed discrimination and marginality as key factors, whereas the later ones expanded the explanations including such cultural factors as assimilation, place identification, and peculiar backgrounds of the subgroups.

Nowadays, scholars seem to agree with the idea "that the differences in recreation preferences stem from values, norms and culture rather than from socio-economic factors" (Andereck et al. 2007, p. 488).

Moreover, it is possible to identify wider connections between the field of cultural psychology and the study of environmental behaviors and perceptions.

The documented differences in attentional patterns (Markus and Kitayama 1991; Masuda and Nisbett 2001), which state that people of Western culture tend to have an analytic perception of the environment whereas people of East Asian culture tend to have a more holistic one, are according to Miyamoto and colleagues (2006) due to the existing differences in the physical environment.

They suggested that the Japanese scenery could be more complex and ambiguous than the American one, *affording* a specific way of perception oriented to the global configuration.

A cultural difference in the aesthetic preferences across cultures has also been stated through the comparison of evaluations of biomes or various landscapes given by samples belonging to different cultural systems.

Ham and colleagues (2004) stated that Chinese participants, compared to the American ones, consistently gave lower preference scores to interiors of greater complexity, researching a higher level of coherence. The same difference was noted about scenes with a vertical design or darkness at the focal point.

The authors concluded that "the findings suggest that preferred and non-preferred environmental design attributes are bounded within a group's cultural experiences" (p. 48).

Han (2007), criticizing a one-dimensional approach to preference centered on an evolutionary explanation, underlined the importance of cultural factors.

He suggested that the American people preferred the coniferous trees because they are relatively common in local parks and backyards.

On the other hand, the Texan students involved gave a high-score evaluation of the tundra biome that was supposed to be attractive in opposition to the humid and hot weather typical of their habitat. Balling and Falk (1982; Falk and Balling 2010) too, while supporting the idea of an innate tendency to prefer savanna, agree with a cultural familiarity having opposite effects on the preference rating.

Herzog and colleagues (2000) stated the cultural variability of the perceived signs of human influence when the Australian members of his sample identified the willow trees seen in landscape pictures as intrusive, not natural, whereas the American participants considered them as part of the natural environment.

Nature as a Positive Experience

Unlike the topic mentioned above and although it is a classic theme in the environmental psychology field, the positive psychological effects triggered by natural environments have been poorly investigated in a cross-cultural perspective.

This happened because the main theories of the field had an evolutionary orientation in attempting to settle the universal processes that can explain the phenomenon and by doing so disregarded the possible cultural variations.

Even if natural benefits are long since known in the popular culture, a first attempt to scientific demonstration of this common understanding was proposed in the psychological field only since the 1970s, with the pioneer works of Kaplan and Kaplan (1978, 1982) and Ulrich (1981, 1984).

In that period in fact, environmental psychology was beginning its transition from an architectonic paradigm to another characterized by a strong attention to nature, proenvironmental behaviors, and sustainability in general.

Currently, a large body of research has shown amply that exposure to natural landscapes has positive effects, such as the promotion of cognitive and emotional development (Wells 2000), individual health and trauma resilience (Ulrich 1984), on individuals on a cross-cultural level.

Hence, several theoretical frameworks give different explanations of how this positive effect is generated.

The main theoretical frameworks, namely, the *Attention Restoration Theory* (Kaplan and Kaplan 1989; Kaplan 1995) and the *Stress Recovery Theory* (Ulrich et al. 1991), tend to explain the environment-well-being relationship as an automatic regulation system, within which people unwittingly regain normal levels of cognitive functioning after a period of mental fatigue.

The *Attention Restoration Theory* was based on two theoretical frameworks, summarized by Kaplan in a biocognitive theory of the man-environment relationship.

The first framework was the seminal work of Berlyne (1950, 1954), stating the evolutionary importance of collative stimuli (novelty, complexity) to help human learning and environmental exploration.

The second was the distinction between voluntary and involuntary attention (James 1892), in which the former is needed to carry on the normal activities of everyday life, often involving a low personal stimulation, and the latter identifies an automatic capture of attention generated by the context of the current activity.

This involvement, which Kaplan called *fascination*, is supposed to be useful as it facilitates the recovery from the fatigue of the directed attention and is favored by the natural context because of our phylogenetic past in a natural world.

Therefore, a restorative place is a landscape full of fascinating features, but at the same time, it is perceived as being very different from the everyday spaces (being away) and compatible with cognitive schemata (compatibility).

Moreover, Korpela (1992) suggested that a higher local restorativeness was correlated to a higher place preference, and that people used the favorite places strategically as "reserves" of cognitive clarity.

The *Stress Recovery Theory* (Ulrich 1984) offered indeed a simpler explanation, adopting the same evolutionary paradigm but suggesting a stress-related approach. In his seminal research, Ulrich tested the postsurgery complications in patients with the same disease but with a different spatial location within the hospital.

Patients with an open view on the inner garden were found to have a shorter recovery time, a decrease in the use of medicines, and a lower emotional stress, in comparison with other patients hospitalized in rooms without views or where they could only watch the wall opposite.

Those results were further extended by the work of Heerwagen and Orians (1986), who found the same effect by using panels with reproductions of nature.

Such a remarkable effect was explained hypothesizing that humans developed a quick automatic response to contents and configurations that "tended to foster survival and well-being" (Ulrich et al. 1991, p. 209) during the phylogenetic evolution of the species.

Moreover, this framework was supposed to explain another consolidated outcome, that is, the major restorative power of natural environments compared with any type of urban area (Kaplan 1987; Staats et al. 2003).

Despite their differences, both Kaplan and Kaplan's and Ulrich's theories focus on restoration; that is to say that they identify the positive effects of nature in facilitating the reaching of an optimal level of functioning.

We can therefore define these theoretical positions as *homeostatic models* as they are both based on a concept of nature as a recovery system with automatic effects on the psychological state, where the focus is on a passive return to a "normal" mental functioning after daily perturbing situations.

On the other hand, recent research proposes alternative views of the nature-wellness relationships, based on the idea that the person-environment relation gives rise to generative processes.

Compared to homeostatic models the main difference is that generative explanations assume that nature actively enhances both an emotional and a cognitive status, generating some *flourishing* effects on subjective skills.

According to Keyes (2002) in fact, to flourish means to experience a condition of perceived well-being and mental health characterized by generativity, personal growth, and resilience.

Moreover, the *Broaden-and-Build Theory* (Fredrickson 2001) stated that experiencing positive emotion could broaden people's momentary thought-action repertoires and, at the same time, build new psychosocial resources available for use in other contexts of daily life.

These flourishing effects should then consist in a rise in system complexity that involves emotional, cognitive, and social abilities, empowered by positive emotions that people experience enjoying natural areas.

Within those *generative models*, several theoretical frameworks hold different mediators as key factors accounting for the positive effect of nature.

Some of the mediators indirectly or directly depend on cultural and social factors.

As mentioned above, Buijs and colleagues (2009) had introduced cultural belonging as a possible explanation of the shared satisfaction about a public natural area.

Some scholars similarly argued that public parks and gardens are socially generative, enhancing community well-being through the reinforcement of relations of proximity (Kuo et al. 1998; Sullivan et al. 2004).

A specific aspect of social mediation is the decreasing incidence of aggressive episodes mediated by the presence of gardens and green areas close to dwellings, due both to a greater informal control, and to positive cognitive effects that attending natural areas can generate (Kuo and Sullivan 2001).

Ryan and collaborators (2010) indicate *subjective vitality* as a possible mediator for the positive effects of nature, representing a significant factor also when controlled for social and physical activity.

Subjective vitality, defined as "one's conscious experience of possessing energy and aliveness" (Ryan and Frederick 1997, p. 530), has also been linked to other indicators of general well-being like positive emotions, satisfaction with life, and self-actualization.

Following a different approach, based on the importance given to the ethical relationship between man and nature, Mayer and McPherson-Frantz (2004) suggested that the psychological benefits of nature are mediated by the sense of *connectedness to nature*, that is, the individual sense of belonging to the natural world.

They also suggested that connectedness is related to some well-being indicators: life satisfaction, eco-friendly behaviors, coping with interpersonal problems.

A similar mediator that should be considered is the *place attachment*, defined as a positive bond that develops between individuals and their social, natural, and built-up environment.

It "involves an interplay of affect and emotions, knowledge and beliefs, and behaviors and actions in reference to a place" (Low and Altman 1992, p. 5).

Place attachments and identities (Proshansky et al. 1983) have been demonstrated to be a secure basis to explore an environment, empowering self-confidence and influencing well-being and healthy self-development in both children and adults; also, they have an identity-definition function. On the other hand, a sudden loss of these bonds caused by natural disasters or intrusions in private territories could provoke negative emotions comparable to those experimented in case of bereavement (Brown and Perkins 1992).

According to Markus and Kitayama (1991), the idea of a place-related identity could have significant points of convergence with the wider concept of "cultural Self," defining the construction of a personal identity as a process depending on cultural and environmental belonging.

Another intervening factor could be traced in the *Flow Theory* (Csikszentmihalyi 1975, 1991). The flow experience has been often cited in environmental psychology because it shares some features with the transcendent and sublime experiences, frequently reported as results of activities in wild nature. Mitchell (1983) underlined two distinct experiences of transcendence in nature, the first one characterized by diminutive feelings of submission and extreme respect and the second marked by subjective well-being and perceived compatibility with the task. Confirming those results, Williams and Harvey (2001) described the *transcendent experience* as characterized by strong positive affects, feeling of overcoming limits, sense of union with the universe or other entities, and sense of being engrossed in the moment and timelessness. Those definitions are close to the main dimensions of the phenomenon of flow of consciousness.

Kaplan and Talbot (1983) added another key similarity, suggesting that the *wilderness experience* produces significant changes in personality traits and a long-term evolution of the cognition-action patterns. In order to avoid states of boredom or anxiety due to the imbalance between environmental challenges and perceived competence, it is necessary for people to experience new and more advanced forms of satisfaction, gradually redefining their self-perception and the thresholds of their perceived optimal balance (Inghilleri 1999, 2003).

Another relevant point of contact can be detected between the flow theory and the idea of fascination. The cognitive clarity (Kaplan and Kaplan 1982), a sensation of cognitive pleasure that arises when people perceive balance between their cognitive schemata and environmental information, is a frequent result during such an experience. That sensation could be easily compared with some features of the flow experience, including a perceived task-skills balance, a strong sense of control, and a focusing of attention without effort.

Also, R. Kaplan (1983) suggested that the attention restoration is not only provoked by the natural context that captures the involuntary attention and facilitates the recovery from the voluntary attention fatigue. Restorative effects are also triggered by a fascination for process. In this case, the focus of attention to the task implies a perceived compatibility between personal capacity and perceived challenges, exactly as it happens when the state of flow is activated.

Moreover, Csikszentmihalyi and Nakamura noted (2010, p. 181):

> When people enjoy most what they are doing—from playing music to playing chess, from reading good books to having a good conversation, from working their best to trying to beat their own record in sport—they report a state of effortless concentration so deep that they lose their sense of time, of themselves, of their problems.

During an optimal experience, the attention flows, then, effortlessly, a definition very similar to that used by James and Kaplan to identify fascination as a form of attention acting without any cognitive effort.

It is interesting to note that this kind of experiences are well known in many traditional cultures. They often characterize the rites of passage, as in the case of the "vision quests" that marked the transition from childhood to adulthood in some Native American traditional celebrations (Inghilleri 1999).

Nature and Well-Being: The Relevance of Culture

Albeit from different theoretical points of reference, the above-mentioned frameworks share some important features.

In fact, they all propose a wider theory about the "green effect," adding new explanations to the evolutionary ones to depict subjects and their autonomy, also involving the sociocultural systems in which they live and act.

Moreover, they all support a vision based on the variability of individual behavior and on multicausality, criticizing the mainstream models for their static and automatic basis, and approach new conceptualizations of "well-being" drawn from the research in positive and cultural psychology.

In brief, it is possible to propose a taxonomy of mediators of nature's benefits:

- *Cognitive mediators (homeostatic):* recovery from stress and mental fatigue
- *Cognitive mediators (generative):* flow experience and self-enhancement
- *Emotional mediators:* connectedness to nature, natural bonding, and place attachment
- *Cultural and social mediators:* belonging to different "interpretive communities," new social relations, and community building

What emerges from this classification is a synergistic presence of genetic, cognitive, and cultural factors that discourages reductionist interpretations centered only on an automatic learning during phylogenesis. It also leads to consider the different factors in a biocultural model so as to build a wider framework.

Some scholars of complex systems (e.g., Monod 1970; Prigogine 1976) and psychologists (Csikszentmihalyi and Massimini 1985; Inghilleri 1999; Massimini and Delle Fave 2000) converge on the hypothesis of the existence of two *teleonomic* projects inside the human species, both aiming for a transgenerational transmission of their specific parts of information.

The first is the biological one, in which genes transmit information to future generations through the mechanisms of Darwinian natural selection.

The second is the cultural one, in which memes (Dawkins 1976) transmit to future generations the information about social rules and meanings, also indicating how to use the artifacts that every system has produced in the course of its evolution. Moreover, both systems interact to guide and direct the subjective behavior (Delle Fave et al. 2011).

The human central nervous system can be considered as a "biocultural entity in which hereditary biological information and internalized and learned cultural information complement each other in order to reproduce genes and memes, or biological and cultural projects" (Inghilleri 1999, p. 15). Consciousness could be then described as a locus where information coming from the natural and the cultural environments interacts with the information coming from the individual, genetic, and cultural internalized instructions (Massimini et al. 1996).

Following this theoretical grid, a natural area could also be defined as an artifact, made of information coming from the evolutionary past, the actual perception, and the cultural heritage simultaneously.

Looking at this model in an ecological perspective (Bronfenbrenner 1977, 1979), the *microsystem* appears to be constituted by the physical reality of an environment, whose positive psychological effects are constructed by interaction with the two superordinate systems.

The first of these, a *mesosystem*, includes some outputs of the process of bio-cultural selection considered to be particularly important in defining "nature" as a historically and geographically grounded artifact. In particular, it comprises shared ethical considerations about the idea of nature in a specific historical moment, social interpretation of nature, individual place attachment and identification, and community dynamics.

The second one represents the wider process of the biocultural selection and the continuous exchange of cultural products between the Self and the cultural system in which it fits.

Differently from Kaplan's theory, this model then proposes that the link between a natural place and an experience of well-being is always mediated by the belonging to a cultural system, in constant dialogue with the phylogenetic information resulting from the history of the species.

This interaction then leads to activate strategic and automatic behaviors in every-day life. As affirmed by Korpela (1992), people tend to make a conscious use of certain places according to their actual cognitive needs. For instance, a natural walk would be more easily chosen when a person needs attention recovery and reflection, as the preference score given to a natural landscape becomes higher if respondents are experiencing a heavier state of mental fatigue (Hartig and Staats 2006).

The described literature suggests the existence of two *environmental strategies* that interact in determining the pleasantness of the experience with nature.

The homeostatic strategy is conductive to cognitive recovery trough attention restoration and stress reduction.

The generative strategy is characterized by an experience of vitality, flow, and positive emotions; it is the trigger for permanent changes in attitudes and behaviors, activating processes of self-enhancement and psychological complexity.

Concluding Remarks

How to preserve, restore, and live our nature is a main theme in contemporary society, and the psychological sciences too are involved in developing strategies to implement a virtuous circle of pleasant environments and quality of life.

This contribution proposes a critical redefinition of the concept of nature for the psychological field, introducing a cultural perspective and connecting different theoretical and methodological approaches.

Agreeing with the statement that "benefits of nature may extend beyond helping people to recover from stress and mental fatigue" (Mayer et al. 2009, p. 609), we suggested that a natural context could be used as a trigger to build self-complexity through meaningful and optimal experiences, and that it could better be defined as an artifact characterized by deep meanings of belonging and connection.

The field of environmental psychology needs to broaden a vision based on an evolutionary framework by starting to consider new causal factors for the well-being in the natural environment.

A significant step forward can be done enlarging the investigation of the subjective experience in the natural context, integrating current knowledge with concepts borrowed from the positive psychology, for instance, the so-called vitality, the flow experience, and the flourishing dynamic.

This process can be useful for understanding how the experience in nature is processed and produces long-term changes in the structure of the Self. The ultimate goal is to define the shared triggers of well-being and consequently to develop techniques and design methods to increase and spread it in society.

Moreover, it is necessary to pay attention to society itself, taking in consideration its shared beliefs, meanings, and the cross-cultural differences. As stated by cultural psychology (Shweder 1991; Inghilleri 2009), behaviors and attitudes are often anchored in a local system of knowledge, also influenced by the forms and the functions of the territory.

Planning a new town, designing a park, or projecting a new building are activities that deal with different *geomentalities*, with deep implications for perceptions, representations, and wishes.

This cultural approach can help scholars and practitioners to avoid the phenomenon of the *cultural parallax* (Nabhan 1995), characterized by the inability to see cultural information and symbolic traces embodied in landscapes, natural, and built-up spaces.

References

Andereck, K., Valentine, K., Vogt, K., & Knopf, R. (2007). A cross-cultural analysis of tourism and quality of life perceptions. *Journal of Sustainable Tourism, 15*(5), 483–502.

Balling, J. D., & Falk, J. H. (1982). Development of visual preference for natural environments. *Environment and Behavior, 14*, 5–28.

Berlyne, D. E. (1950). Novelty and curiosity as determinants of exploratory behavior. *British Journal of Psychology, 41*(12), 68–80.

Berlyne, D. E. (1954). A theory of human curiosity. *British Journal of Psychology, 45*(3), 180–191.

Berry, J. W. (1980). Acculturation as varieties of adaptation. In A. Padilla (Ed.), *Acculturation: Theory, models and some new findings* (pp. 9–25). Boulder: Westview.

Bronfenbrenner, U. (1977). Toward an experimental ecology of human development. *American Psychologist, 32*(7), 513–531.

Bronfenbrenner, U. (1979). *The ecology of human development: Experiments by nature and design.* Cambridge: Harvard University Press.

Brown, B., & Perkins, D. D. (1992). Disruptions in place attachment. In I. Altman & S. M. Low (Eds.), *Place attachment* (pp. 279–304). New York: Plenum Press.

Buijs, A. E., Elands, B. H. M., & Langers, F. (2009). No wilderness for immigrants: Cultural differences in images of nature and landscape preferences. *Landscape and Urban Planning, 91*(3), 113–123.

Byrne, J., & Wolch, J. (2009). Nature, race, and parks: Past research and future directions for geographic research. *Progress in Human Geography, 33*(6), 743–765.

Chavez, D. J. (2001). *Managing outdoor recreation in California: Visitor contact studies 1989–1998 (General Technical Report PSW-GTR-180).* Albany: USDA Forest Service, Pacific Southwest Research Station.

Csikszentmihalyi, M. (1975). *Beyond boredom and anxiety.* San Francisco: Jossey-Bass.

Csikszentmihalyi, M. (1991). *Flow: The psychology of optimal experience: Steps toward enhancing the quality of life.* New York: Harper Collins.

Csikszentmihalyi, M., & Massimini, F. (1985). On the psychological selection of bio-cultural information. *New Ideas in Psychology, 3*(2), 115–138.

Csikszentmihalyi, M., & Nakamura, J. (2010). Effortless attention in everyday life: A systematic phenomenology. In B. Bruya (Ed.), *Effortless attention: A new perspective in the cognitive science of attention and action* (pp. 179–190). Cambridge: MIT Press.

Dawkins, R. (1976). *The selfish gene.* Oxford: Oxford University Press.

Delle Fave, A., Massimini, F., & Bassi, M. (2011). *Psychological selection and optimal experience across cultures.* New York: Springer.

Ehlers, E. (2003). Environment across culture: An introduction. In C. F. Gethmann & E. Ehlers (Eds.), *Environment across cultures* (pp. 1–9). Berlin: Springer.

Falk, J. H., & Balling, J. D. (2010). Evolutionary influence on human landscape preference. *Environment and Behavior, 42,* 479–493.

Floyd, M. F., Bocarro, J. N., & Thompson, T. (2008). Research on race and ethnicity in leisure studies: A review of five major journals. *Journal of Leisure Research, 40*(1), 1–22.

Fredrickson, B. L. (2001). The role of positive emotions in positive psychology: The broaden-and-build theory of positive emotions. *American Psychologist, 56,* 218–226.

Gesler, W. (1996). Lourdes: Healing in a place of pilgrimage. *Health & Place, 2,* 95–105.

Ham, T. Y., Guerin, D. A., & Scott, S. C. (2004). A cross-cultural comparison of preference for visual attributes in interior environments: America and China. *Journal of Interior Design, 30*(2), 37–50.

Han, K. T. (2007). Responses to six major terrestrial biomes in terms of scenic beauty, preference, and restorativeness. *Environment and Behavior, 39,* 529–556.

Hartig, T., & Staats, H. (2006). The need for psychological restoration as a determinant of environmental preferences. *Journal of Environmental Psychology, 26*(3), 215–226.

Heerwagen, J. H., & Orians, G. H. (1986). Adaptations to windowlessness: A study of the use of visual decor in windowed and windowless offices. *Environment and Behavior, 18*(5), 623–639.

Herzog, T. R., Herbert, E. J., Kaplan, R., & Crooks, C. L. (2000). Cultural and developmental comparisons of landscape perceptions and preferences. *Environment and Behavior, 32,* 323–346.

Inghilleri, P. (1999). *From subjective experience to cultural change.* Cambridge: Cambridge University Press.

Inghilleri, P. (2003). *La buona vita: Per l'uso creativo degli oggetti nella società dell'abbondanza.* Milano: Guerini & Associati.

Inghilleri, P. (Ed.). (2009). *Psicologia culturale.* Milano: Raffaello Cortina Editore.

James, W. (1892). *Psychology: The briefer course.* New York: Holt.

Kaplan, R. (1983). The role of nature in the urban context. In I. Altman & J. F. Wohlwill (Eds.), *Behavior and the natural environment* (pp. 127–161). New York: Plenum Press.

Kaplan, S. (1987). Aesthetics, affect and cognition: Environmental preference from an evolutionary perspective. *Environment and Behavior, 19,* 3–32.

Kaplan, S. (1995). The restorative benefits of nature: Toward an integrative framework. *Journal of Environmental Psychology, 15*(3), 169–182.

Kaplan, R., & Kaplan, S. (1978). *Humanscape: Environments for people.* North Scituate: Duxbury Press.

Kaplan, S., & Kaplan, R. (1982). *Cognition and environment: Functioning in an uncertain world.* New York: Praeger.

Kaplan, R., & Kaplan, S. (1989). *The experience of nature: A psychological perspective.* New York: Cambridge University Press.

Kaplan, S., & Talbot, J. F. (1983). Psychological benefits of a wilderness experience. In I. Altman & J. F. Wohlwill (Eds.), *Behavior and the natural environment* (pp. 163–203). New York: Plenum Press.

Kaplan, R., & Talbot, J. F. (1988). Ethnicity and preference for natural settings: A review and recent findings. *Landscape and Urban Planning, 15*, 107–117.

Kellert, S. R. (1995). Concepts of nature east and west. In M. E. Soulé & G. Lease (Eds.), *Reinventing nature?: Responses to postmodern deconstruction* (pp. 103–121). Washington, DC: Island Press.

Keyes, C. L. (2002). The mental health continuum: From languishing to flourishing in life. *Journal of Health and Social Behavior, 43*, 207–222.

Kluckhohn, F. R., & Strodtbeck, F. (1961). *Variations in value orientations.* New York: Row Peterson.

Korpela, K. (1992). Adolescents favorite places and environmental self-regulation. *Journal of Environmental Psychology, 9*, 241–256.

Kuo, F. E., & Sullivan, W. C. (2001). Environment and crime in the inner city. *Environment and Behavior, 33*, 343–367.

Kuo, F. E., Sullivan, W. C., Coley, R. L., & Brunson, L. (1998). Fertile ground for community: Inner-city neighborhood common spaces. *American Journal of Community Psychology, 26*(6), 823–851.

Low, S. M., & Altman, I. (1992). Place attachment: A conceptual inquiry. In I. Altman & S. M. Low (Eds.), *Place attachment* (pp. 1–12). New York: Plenum Press.

Markus, H. R., & Kitayama, S. (1991). Culture and the self: Implications for cognition, emotion and motivation. *Psychological Review, 98*(2), 224–253.

Massimini, F., & Delle Fave, A. (2000). Individual development in a bio-cultural perspective. *American Psychologist, 55*(1), 24–33.

Massimini, F., Inghilleri, P., & Delle, F. A. (1996). *La selezione psicologica umana: Teoria e metodo d'analisi.* Milano: Cooperativa Libraria IULM.

Masuda, T., & Nisbett, R. E. (2001). Attending holistically vs. analytically: Comparing the context sensitivity of Japanese and Americans. *Journal of Personality and Social Psychology, 81*, 922–934.

Mayer, F. S., & McPherson-Frantz, C. (2004). The connectedness to nature scale: A measure of individuals' feeling in community with nature. *Journal of Environmental Psychology, 24*(4), 503–515.

Mayer, F. S., McPherson-Frantz, C., Bruehlman-Senecal, E., & Dolliver, K. (2009). Why is nature beneficial?: The role of connectedness to nature. *Environment and Behavior, 41*(5), 607–643.

Merchant, N. (2003). *Reinventing Eden: The fate of nature in western culture.* London: Routledge.

Minteer, B. A., & Manning, R. E. (1999). Pragmatism in environmental ethics: Democracy, pluralism, and the management of nature. *Environmental Ethics, 21*, 191–208.

Mitchell, R. G. (1983). *Mountain experience: The psychology and sociology of adventure.* Chicago: University of Chicago Press.

Miyamoto, Y., Nisbett, R. E., & Masuda, T. (2006). Culture and the physical environment: Holistic versus analytic perceptual affordances. *Psychological Science, 17*, 113–119.

Monod, J. (1970). *Le hasard et la nécessité.* Paris: Éditions du Seuil.

Nabhan, G. P. (1995). Cultural parallax in viewing North American habitats. In M. E. Soulé & G. Lease (Eds.), *Reinventing nature?: Responses to postmodern deconstruction* (pp. 87–101). Washington: Island Press.

Nash, R. (1967). *Wilderness and the American mind.* New Haven: Yale University Press.

Prigogine, I. (1976). Order through fluctuation: Self-organization and social system. In E. Jantsch & L. H. Waddington (Eds.), *Evolution and consciousness: Human systems in transition* (pp. 93–133). Reading: Addison-Wesley.

Proshansky, H. M., Fabian, A. K., & Kaminoff, R. (1983). Place identity: Physical social world organization of the self. *Journal of Environmental Psychology, 3*, 57–83.

Redclift, M. (2003). Sustainability discourses: Human livelihoods and life chances. In C. F. Gethmann & E. Ehlers (Eds.), *Environment across cultures* (pp. 175–183). Berlin: Springer.

Ryan, R. M., & Frederick, C. (1997). On energy, personality, and health: Subjective vitality as a dynamic reflection of well-being. *Journal of Personality, 65,* 529–566.

Ryan, R. M., Weinstein, N., Bernstein, J. H., Brown, K. W., Mistretta, L., & Gagné, M. (2010). Vitalizing effects of being outdoors and in nature. *Journal of Environmental Psychology, 30*(2), 159–168.

Shweder, R. A. (1991). *Thinking trough cultures: Expeditions in cultural psychology.* Cambridge: Harvard University Press.

Sieferle, P. (2003). The ends of nature. In C. F. Gethmann & E. Ehlers (Eds.), *Environment across cultures* (pp. 13–28). Berlin: Springer.

Staats, H., Kieviet, A., & Hartig, T. (2003). Where to recover from attentional fatigue: An expectancy-value analysis of environmental preference. *Journal of Environmental Psychology, 23,* 147–157.

Sullivan, W. C., Kuo, F. E., & Depooter, S. F. (2004). The fruit of urban nature. *Environment and Behavior, 36*(5), 678–700.

Ulrich, R. S. (1981). Natural versus urban scenes: Some psychophysiological effects. *Environment and Behavior, 13,* 523–556.

Ulrich, R. S. (1984). View through window may influence recovery from surgery. *Science, 224,* 420–421.

Ulrich, R. S., Simons, R., Losito, B., Fiorito, E., Miles, M., & Zelson, M. (1991). Stress recovery during exposure to natural and urban environments. *Journal of Environmental Psychology, 11*(3), 201–230.

Von Glasersfeld, E. (1984). An introduction to radical constructivism. In P. Watzlawick (Ed.), *The invented reality* (pp. 17–40). New York: Norton.

Vygotskij, L. S. (1934/1962). *Thought and speech.* Cambridge: MIT Press.

Wells, N. M. (2000). At home with nature: Effects of greenness on children's cognitive functioning. *Environment and Behavior, 32,* 775–795.

Williams, K., & Harvey, D. (2001). Transcendent experience in forest environments. *Journal of Environmental Psychology, 21*(3), 249–260.

Yoon, H. (2003). A preliminary attempt to give a birdseye view on the nature of traditional eastern (Asian) and western (European) environmental ideas. In C. F. Gethmann & E. Ehlers (Eds.), *Environment across cultures* (pp. 123–142). Berlin: Springer.

Chapter 8
Religion, Spirituality, and Well-Being Across Nations: The Eudaemonic and Hedonic Happiness Investigation

Antonella Delle Fave, Ingrid Brdar, Dianne Vella-Brodrick, and Marie P. Wissing

Introduction

The interest of academic psychology in religion and spirituality is relatively recent. Although, for several years dedicated journals and books have been published on these topics, the vast majority of scientific publications in psychology have dealt only marginally with such topics. A special issue of the Personality and Social Psychology Review, opening with an editorial titled "Why does religiosity persist?" (Sedikides 2010) recently attempted to explain the reasons for this gap in the psychological literature, providing a general overview of the theories and approaches currently available to investigate religiousness and related topics. The picture concerning quality of life and well-being research is, however, different with the number of studies investigating the relationship between religiousness/spirituality and physical and mental health steadily increasing.

In this chapter, we will present some international findings on the perception of happiness and meaningfulness in the spirituality/religion domain. Before showing our results, however, we will briefly summarize the main research advancements in this field.

A. Delle Fave (✉)
Dipartimento di Scienze Cliniche Luigi Sacco, Università degli Studi di Milano, Milan, Italy
e-mail: antonella.dellefave@unimi.it

I. Brdar
Faculty of Humanities & Social Sciences, University of Rijeka, Rijeka, Croatia

D. Vella-Brodrick
School of Psychology and Psychiatry, Monash University, Melbourne, Australia

M.P. Wissing
School for Psychosocial Behavioural Sciences, North-West University, Potchefstroom, South Africa

H.H. Knoop and A. Delle Fave (eds.), *Well-Being and Cultures: Perspectives from Positive Psychology*, Cross-Cultural Advancements in Positive Psychology 3, DOI 10.1007/978-94-007-4611-4_8, © Springer Science+Business Media Dordrecht 2013

Religiousness and Spirituality: Definition Challenges

Spirituality was variously described as a subjective experience of sacredness and transcendence (Vaughan 1991), the search for and the construction of an existential meaning (Bellingham et al. 1989; King et al. 1995), a contact with the divine within the self (Fahlberg and Fahlberg 1991), and the feeling of connectedness and integration – with a transcendent power, with oneself, with nature, with one's community. Recently, van Dierendonck (2011) explored it within the framework of self-determination theory, suggesting spirituality be considered as a basic psychological need.

The term religiousness refers instead to the participation in a belief system which comprises specific and institutionalized values, norms, and rituals (O'Collins and Farrugia 1991; King et al. 2001). The pioneer work by Allport and Ross (1967) pointed to the need for investigating religiousness according to its meaning and role for individuals, drawing a distinction between intrinsic religiosity – referring to the personal identification with a belief system – and extrinsic religiosity – instrumentally used to cope with distress or to get social support. Subsequent studies highlighted that these two aspects are often combined in the individual experience of religiousness. Religion includes a complex set of behavioral rules providing individuals with short-term and long-term opportunities for action and goal setting (Emmons 2005, 2006). It offers an explanatory perspective of the human existence, thus supporting the process of meaning making and allowing individuals to transcend their own limited self toward a wider vision of reality (Sperry and Shafranske 2005). This process is influenced both by the cultural and religious context and by personal predispositions, life experiences, and the hierarchy of priorities and values that individuals ceaselessly build and shape throughout their lives.

This brief overview suggests that spirituality and religiousness share conceptual/ experiential similarities, as well as differences, which are further related to the cultural context in which they are evaluated. Some scholars have expressed their concerns about the methodological and interpretive consequences of this partial overlapping for research. For example, Koenig (2008) recently argued that most of the scales currently used to assess spirituality substantially investigate positive psychological traits and behaviors, such as gratitude, forgiveness, peace of mind, purpose in life, and meaning, thus hindering the identification of authentically religious dimensions. However, although an increasing number of people – especially in Western countries – define themselves as spiritual but not as religious, the majority of people who report being religious also define themselves as spiritual (Joshanloo 2010; Shahabi et al. 2002). Moreover, due to the multifaceted contents of the two terms, and their strong interconnection, the joint assessment of spirituality and religiousness through items and scales simultaneously evaluating the two dimensions can provide researchers with valuable information (Tsuang and Simpson 2008; Tiliouine 2009; Wills 2009). This is particularly true of cross-cultural studies, in which findings are gathered in social contexts widely varying in terms of importance attributed to each of these two dimensions.

Religiousness, Spirituality, and Well-Being

The importance of evaluating religiousness and spirituality among indicators of quality of life is confirmed by the vast literature on well-being. In particular, several studies emphasized the benefits of religiousness for both mental and physical health (Myers 2000). In a broad review of the literature, Koenig and his colleagues (2001) showed that 79% of the studies conducted on this topic highlighted a significant and positive relationship between religiousness and well-being. The stability of this relationship was systematically confirmed by longitudinal studies.

Epidemiological analyses revealed a positive correlation between religious practice and low incidence of cardiovascular diseases, cancer, and mortality in general (Larson et al. 1989; McCullough et al. 2000). This relationship was ascribed to aspects of religion substantially related to the promotion of positive psychological features and mental health (Mytko and Knight 1999): most religious systems prescribe healthy lifestyles and food habits; prayer and meditation foster psychophysical relaxation; religious practice provides social support through participation in community rituals and activities; religiousness fosters the perception of meaning, optimism, hope, and a more active acceptance of negative events (Bickel et al. 1998; Brady et al. 1999; Jenkins and Pargament 1995; Park 2005; Spiegel and Fawzy 2002). The multifaceted role of religiousness in promoting well-being under stressful circumstances was confirmed in both cross-sectional and longitudinal studies involving participants facing terminal illness or bereavement (McClain et al. 2003; Walsh et al. 2002).

More recently, a meta-analysis of published studies evaluating the association between religiosity/spirituality and mortality (Chida et al. 2009) detected the protective role of organizational activities connected to religion (such as church attendance) for the survival of healthy populations. Chida and colleagues however pointed to the mediating role of other biopsychosocial factors related to religion and identified in previous studies, such as family lifestyle, stress buffering, social support, promotion of life satisfaction, and positive emotions (Ano and Vasconcelles 2005; Fredrickson 2002; Gillum and Ingram 2006; Howell et al. 2007). These empirical findings show that spirituality and religion are related to most of the well-being dimensions currently investigated in positive psychology. However, their prominent connections seem to emerge with eudaemonic aspects, such as meaning making, self-actualization, the pursuit of virtues, and self-transcendence.

Religiousness, Spirituality, and Culture

The relevance of religion and spirituality in providing people with individual and collective meanings and values are widely acknowledged (Emmons and McCullough 2004; Geyer and Baumeister 2005; McCullough et al. 2000). However, meanings, together with religious beliefs and spirituality themselves, stem from culture.

They are components of the cultural network in which individuals grow and develop their talents and potentials (Massimini and Delle Fave 1991). This represent a crucial challenge for researchers, as most studies on religion and spirituality were previously conducted in Western countries, characterized by the Judaic-Christian tradition, with its specific implications for daily behavior and relationship with the divine (Paloutzian and Park 2005; Sperry and Shafranske 2005). Although some empirical findings showed cultural differences in levels of spirituality and religiousness in an African context (e.g., Burnell et al. 2009; Patel et al. 2009), a much broader cross-cultural perspective is needed to understand the psychological and psychosocial roles of religiousness and spirituality (Tarakeshwar et al. 2003).

The first international contribution toward this aim was provided within the framework of quality of life (QoL) research (WHOQOL Group 2006). Religion and spirituality were investigated as components of quality of life, defined by WHO as the individuals' perception of their position and role in their own life, culture, and value system, taking into account their personal expectations and goals. The domains identified as core components of QoL were physical health, psychological dimensions, independence, social relations, and environment, as well as spirituality, religion, and personal beliefs. Data gathered in 18 different countries showed that religion and spirituality play an independent role in influencing perceived quality of life across cultures.

Other studies confirmed the independent contribution of spirituality to general well-being indicators in different cultures. The specific contribution of religion and spirituality to well-being was highlighted by Wills (2009), who conducted a survey in Colombia integrating the Personal Well-Being Index (PWI; Cummins et al. 2004) with an additional item evaluating satisfaction with spirituality/religiosity. Findings suggested the need for including this dimension as a separate domain in the PWI. Similar evidence was obtained by Tiliouine (2009) in Algeria. Other studies, however, provided discrepant findings, showing a very modest contribution of religiosity/spirituality to the general level of well-being and happiness in a variety of countries such as Pakistan, Norway, Denmark, and the USA (Abdel-Khalek 2006; Snoep 2008; Suhail and Chaudry 2004; Tsuang et al. 2007).

In contrast with this increasing number of international statistical surveys on religious belief and practice, very few studies have examined the role of spirituality and religiousness by means of findings indirectly obtained through the analysis of daily time budget and through qualitative instruments investigating daily experience and long-term projects. These procedures allow participants to freely report their priorities, goals, and values – among them religion and spirituality – without being forced to focus on these specific dimensions through ad hoc research questions. This approach can thus offer a different perspective on the role of religion and spirituality in participants' life. Within this framework, a study was conducted on 870 adult participants, belonging to both Western (59.3%) and non-Western cultures (40.7%), in order to investigate the occurrence of optimal experience (or *flow*) and associated activities in their lives (Delle Fave et al. 2011a). When invited to indicate their religion in the demographic section of the questionnaire, most participants easily identified it, and – especially in non-Western countries – they reported to regularly perform individual prayer and rituals. However, while the vast majority reported optimal experience in their lives, only 5.6% of the participants (most of them from non-Western countries) associated it with spirituality and religious practice. An even lower percentage of participants referred to religion and spirituality when invited to list their main present challenges and future goals.

Totally different findings were obtained among people who had intentionally chosen to cultivate religion as a prominent activity of their daily life. Findings obtained from Italian religious participants belonging to various Catholic orders and congregations and lay members of Catholic associations (Coppa and Delle Fave 2007, 2009) showed that 81.2% of the consecrated people and 58.6% of the lay practicing people associated optimal experience with religious practice (mainly referring to individual prayer and contemplation). Religion was also prominent among their present challenges, in terms of coherence between behavior and religious ideals, effort to overcome egoism and selfishness, and development of a personal relationship with God. Similar findings were obtained from Spanish religious and lay practicing participants (Zaccagnini et al. 2010).

These results can be better interpreted if we consider religious belief systems as components of the cultural milieu in which people grow and develop their talents and potentials (Delle Fave et al. 2011a). Cultivation of religious and spiritual practices are not necessarily challenges or goals per se, but rather they play a background role, orienting individuals' identity development, value system, and the pursuit of meaningful challenges and goals. However, when actively selected by the individuals as core components of their daily life and developmental trajectory, spirituality and religion can become prominent opportunities for flow and lifelong commitment.

In Western cultures, as highlighted by Zinnbauer and Pargament (2005), the rise in popularity of the concept of spirituality, together with the decline of traditional religious practices and institutions, produced a tendency to juxtapose the two constructs in positive versus negative terms. While spirituality is currently perceived as dynamic, functional to the search for existential meanings, rooted in the subjective experience of transcendence, and thus authentic and personalized, religion is described as a static and institutionalized system of prescriptions and dogmas that constrains the individual into well-defined pathways. As a matter of fact in most Western countries, characterized by a Christian tradition, during the past decades religious practice and commitment declined, leaving room to agnosticism or to other forms of spirituality, often related to Asian traditions (The Association of Religion Data Archives 2009). Recent surveys (NationMaster 2010) showed that, with the exceptions of Poland and Ireland, in European countries only a minority of citizens report to attend church, with percentages ranging from 4% in Iceland to 47% in Portugal. In line with these findings, Diener et al. (2011) detected a relationship between religiousness and societal circumstances: compared with highly developed nations, in countries with more difficult life conditions, a higher percentage of people report being religious, and religiousness is associated with higher levels of subjective well-being.

Aims of This Chapter

Based on the theoretical assumptions and empirical evidence reported in the previous sections, this chapter aims to explore the ratings of perceived happiness and meaningfulness in the spirituality/religiousness life domain across seven countries. We also attempted to identify groups of individuals with similar profiles of spiritual/ religious happiness and meaningfulness and to compare the overall levels of well-being of these groups across countries. In line with the prevailing conceptual approach reported in the previous pages, participants were invited to concurrently evaluate spirituality and religiosity with regard to their perceived level of happiness and level of meaningfulness. The data collected on this topic were included in a wider research project aimed at analyzing some of the components of well-being: the Hedonic and Eudaimonic Happiness Investigation.

The Eudaemonic and Hedonic Happiness Investigation: Spirituality/Religiousness and Well-Being

Participants and Research Instruments

Homogeneous subgroups of participants from seven countries and three continents took part (Australia, Croatia, Germany, Italy, Portugal, Spain, South Africa, $N = 666$). Subgroups per country were homogeneous in the sense that they included participants in the adult developmental phase of life and were balanced according to gender, age, and educational level. The subsample per country included equal numbers in the age categories of 30–40 and 41–51, equal numbers of participants with secondary or tertiary level educational qualifications in each age category, and equal numbers of male and female participants at each educational level. All participants were recruited purposively in urban areas according to the specified selection criteria, and with implementation of the snowball method of participant selection. Most participants were employed (91.1%), the majority were married or cohabited with a stable partner (59% and 12.2%, respectively), most participants had children (66.2%), and the majority were Christians (70.8%). See Delle Fave et al. (2011b) for further details on participants and procedures.

Data were collected with the Eudaimonic and Hedonic Investigation instrument (EHHI). The EHHI evaluates lay people's conceptualizations and experiences of happiness, meaningfulness, and goals (see Delle Fave et al. 2011b, for details), adopting a mixed method approach. A short sociodemographic questionnaire was also administered to collect information on participants' gender, age, level of education, work, standard of living, marital status, number of children, religion, and hobbies.

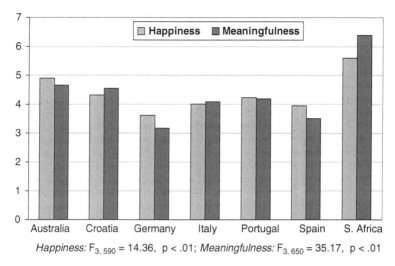

Happiness: $F_{3, 590}$ = 14.36, p < .01; Meaningfulness: $F_{3, 650}$ = 35.17, p < .01

Fig. 8.1 Happiness and meaningfulness in spiritual life domain across the countries

For the purposes of this chapter, we will refer to a subset of the quantitative data collected through the EHHI. In particular, we will refer to data collected with two 7-point rating scales measuring the degree of happiness and degree of experienced meaningfulness in spirituality/religiousness as a life domain (other domains of life explored were work, family, standard of living, interpersonal relationships, health, personal growth, society issues, community issues, leisure, and life in general).

Results

Happiness and Meaningfulness in Spirituality/Religion Across Countries

There was a significant difference among countries in happiness experienced in the spiritual domain (Fig. 8.1). The highest level of happiness was found in the South African sample, and Australian participants reported the second highest mean happiness ratings for spirituality. Participants from these countries differed significantly from the German participants who experienced the lowest level of happiness in the spiritual life domain.

Meaning assigned to spirituality also differed significantly across countries. South Africans reported the highest values of meaning in the domain of spirituality/religion, while German and Spanish participants scored lowest.

In the demographic section of the EHHI, participants were asked to report their religion. The number of participants providing a positive answer varied across countries (chi-square = 63.69, $p < .01$). Portuguese and South African samples had the highest number of religious participants, while the German sample, followed by the Australian sample, comprised the highest number of nonreligious participants (Table 8.1).

Table 8.1 Distribution of
religious and nonreligious
participants across the
countries

Country	Religion		
	No (%)	Yes (%)	N
Australia	36.7	63.3	98
Croatia	14.4	85.6	97
Germany	42.2	57.8	83
Italy	15.2	84.8	92
Portugal	6.0	94.0	67
Spain	27.2	72.8	92
South Africa	6.9	93.1	101
Total	21.4	78.6	630

Table 8.2 Cluster centers on spiritual happiness and meaningfulness

	Clusters				
	High	Happy	Meaning	Low	
Variables	N=231	N=151	N=80	N=127	$F_{3,585}^{a}$
Happiness	6	5	3	2	703.22**
Meaningfulness	6	4	5	2	972.23**

**$p < .01$
^{a}All differences between groups are significant at the .05 level (Student-Newman-Keuls test)

Profiles of Happiness and Meaningfulness in the Spirituality/ Religiousness Domain

The second aim of the present study was to explore whether participants can be classified into groups according to their happiness and meaningfulness in the spiritual domain. Four clusters were identified by K-means cluster analysis (Table 8.2). Two of these groups which are labeled as *High* and *Low* clusters include participants with the highest and lowest ratings respectively on both variables (happiness and meaningfulness). The *Happy* cluster comprises participants who assigned more happiness than meaning to the spiritual domain, while the *Meaning* cluster is composed of participants with higher ratings of meaningfulness than happiness.

The clusters were differently distributed across the countries (chi-square = 157.34, $p < .01$). The great majority of South Africans (84.6%) were included in the *High* cluster (Table 8.3). Participants in German, Portuguese, and Spanish samples were more or less equally distributed across three clusters, with the lowest number of participants in the *Meaning* cluster. Most Australians were distributed in two clusters, *Happy* and *High*, with the highest number of participants placed in the *Meaning* cluster (compared with other countries). Most Italian participants fell into two clusters, *High* and *Low*, with equal number (34.4%).

The number of religious and nonreligious participants differed across clusters (chi-square = 23.13, $p < .01$). Almost half of religious participants (43.1%) fell in the *High* cluster (Table 8.4), while the *Low* cluster comprised the highest number of nonreligious participants (36.5%).

Table 8.3 Distribution of spiritual clusters across the countries

Country		High	Happy	Meaning	Low	Total
		Clusters				
Australia	N	29	33	19	9	90
	%	32.2	36.7	21.1	10.0	100
Croatia	N	32	22	19	18	91
	%	35.2	24.2	20.9	19.8	100
Germany	N	12	20	3	25	60
	%	20.0	33.3	5.0	41.7	100
Italy	N	32	16	13	32	93
	%	34.4	17.2	14.0	34.4	100
Portugal	N	20	26	8	20	74
	%	27.0	35.1	10.8	27.0	100
Spain	N	18	25	12	22	77
	%	23.4	32.5	15.6	28.6	100
South Africa	N	88	9	6	1	104
	%	84.6	8.7	5.8	1.0	100
Total	N	231	151	80	127	589
	%	39.2	25.6	13.6	21.6	100

Table 8.4 Relative frequency of religious and nonreligious participants across clusters

Religion	High	Happy	Meaning	Low	N
	Clusters				
No (%)	24.0	28.1	11.5	36.5	96
Yes (%)	43.1	25.8	14.3	16.8	469
Total (%)	39.8	26.2	13.8	20.2	565

Well-Being Across Clusters and Countries

We hypothesized that happiness and meaningfulness in the spiritual/religious domain would contribute to general well-being. Three measures of well-being were compared among four clusters and across countries: (1) satisfaction with life, (2) happiness in general, and (3) meaningfulness in general. Since religiosity might be correlated with a person's happiness and meaningfulness in the spiritual life domain, analyses of covariance were performed, with religiosity as a covariate.

As Table 8.5 shows, participants in the *High* cluster were more satisfied with their lives and experienced more meaning in general when compared with participants in other clusters. With respect to happiness in general, participants in both *High* and *Happy* clusters reported experiencing higher happiness than participants from the other two clusters. Participants in the *Low* cluster reported the least meaning in general.

Findings also highlighted some country differences in meaningfulness in general (Fig. 8.2). Australian participants, who were significantly more satisfied with their

Table 8.5 Well-being of participants with different profiles of happiness and meaningfulness across countries

Well-being	Country	Clusters High (1)	Happy (2)	Meaning (3)	Low (4)	F (ANCOVA)[a] Clusters	Country	Clusters × country	Post hoc[b]
Satisfaction with life	Australia	5.54	5.17	5.16	4.42	10.48**	4.39**	1.55	*Clusters:* 1–3,4; 2–3
	Croatia	4.86	4.60	4.45	4.42				
	Germany	4.92	5.17	3.33	4.93				*Country:* Australia – Croatia, Italy, Portugal; Italy – Spain
	Italy	5.10	4.29	4.02	4.17				
	Portugal	5.17	4.67	3.88	4.28				
	Spain	4.69	5.35	4.73	4.72				
	South Africa	5.08	4.67	4.23	3.60				
Happiness in general	Australia	5.76	5.61	5.00	4.67	11.17**	1.05	0.81	*Clusters:* 1,2–3,4
	Croatia	5.56	5.36	5.00	5.33				
	Germany	5.67	5.74	5.00	5.08				
	Italy	5.78	5.38	4.69	4.90				
	Portugal	5.60	5.15	4.88	4.95				
	Spain	5.44	5.88	5.08	5.19				
	South Africa	5.52	5.33	4.83	4.00				
Meaning in general	Australia	5.97	5.52	5.84	4.89	12.56**	4.17*	2.10**	*Clusters:* 1–2; 1,2,3–4
	Croatia	6.50	5.95	6.00	6.00				
	Germany	6.40	6.30	4.67	5.20				*Country:* Australia – Croatia, Italy, Spain
	Italy	6.53	5.75	6.23	5.71				
	Portugal	5.95	5.69	6.63	5.60				
	Spain	6.06	5.88	6.67	5.55				
	South Africa	6.22	5.33	5.33	4.00				

$**p < .01$; $*p < .05$

[a]Controlled for religion (no – yes). The covariate was not significant for either of well-being variables. Degrees of freedom: for clusters – 3,585; for country – 6,585; for interaction – 18,585

[b]Sidak adjustment for multiple comparisons

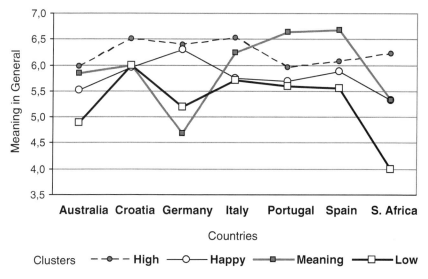

Fig. 8.2 Meaning in general across clusters and countries

Table 8.6 Correlation between happiness and meaningfulness in spirituality/religiousness across countries

Country	r
Australia	.36**
Croatia	.74**
Germany	.94**
Italy	.77**
Portugal	.85**
Spain	.86**
South Africa	.41**

**p < .01

lives than participants from Croatia, Italy, and Portugal, also reported higher values of meaning in general than Croatian, Italian, and Spanish participants. Interestingly, South Africans had the largest difference in meaning in general among clusters, whereas in the Croatian sample, this difference was the smallest. Also, only South Africans included in *Happy* and *Meaning* clusters experienced the same level of meaningfulness in general.

These findings suggest the need to also take into account the relationship between happiness and meaningfulness in the spiritual/religious domain, as they represent two distinct aspects of well-being. As shown in Table 8.6, the correlation between the two variables varied widely across countries.

Discussion

The first aim of this study was to examine if there were differences in happiness and meaningfulness ratings across the seven countries on the spiritual/religious domain. As predicted, significant differences across the countries were found. Participants from South Africa and Australia reported the highest levels of spiritual happiness and meaning, while those from Germany reported the lowest ones. When participants' reported affiliation to a specific religion was examined, Portugal and South Africa had the highest percentage of participants who reported being affiliation. In contrast, German and Australian participants reported affiliation to a religion in the lowest percentage. The findings did not highlight any clear association between spiritual happiness and meaningfulness and religious affiliation, with some countries being high on both (South Africa), others being low on both (Germany), some being moderate on both (Italy), and others still being high on one aspect but low on the other (Australia). However, as suggested by Tarakeshwar et al. (2003), the cultural context may be an important factor in understanding these varied associations between spirituality ratings and religious affiliation.

The comparison between spirituality/religiousness meaning and happiness ratings with the percentage of religious people for each country provided some interesting findings, which support the notion that religion is perceived to be strongly associated with spirituality, but spirituality need not be associated with religion. This is most evident for the South African and Australian data; the two countries with the highest ratings on happiness and meaning in the spiritual/religious domain. A high percentage of South Africans reported being religious (93.1%) and also expressed high levels of spiritual happiness and meaning. Hence, South African participants may equate religion with spirituality and/or vice versa. This interpretation is consistent with Eckersley's (2007) remark that spirituality is most commonly represented via religion which typically involves an institutionalized process of worshipping a higher being. This perspective is also consistent with findings indicating that those who consider themselves religious also tend to report being spiritual (Joshanloo 2010; Shahabi et al. 2002). An alternative explanation may be that South Africans incorporate into their lives high levels of both religiousness and spirituality, perceived as two separate constructs which are developed through different mechanisms and behaviors. However, the former explanation is more probable. In a South African context, both spirituality and religiosity translate into being "a believer" in a greater power. Spirituality and religiosity are intertwined, as expressed by a South African in an interview: "*I cannot live without the idea of God. I experience my spirituality in my struggle with my religion.*"

Importantly, it is possible that in countries with *low* percentages of religious people high numbers of individuals nevertheless report high levels of spiritual happiness and meaningfulness. Australia is a case in point, having the second highest rating for spiritual/religious happiness and meaning and the second *lowest* percentage of people reporting to belong to a religion. This is consistent with the findings of Peach (2003) who noted that less than a quarter of Australians attend church at least monthly. In Australia, as is the case across many Western countries, religion has become less popular, while spirituality has increased in popularity (Bouma 2006; Zinnbauer and Pargament 2005). This is thought to be related to the negative connotations many Australians have about religion being associated with formal organizations (Bouma 2006). Australians generally derive considerably more meaning from nature and their environment than they do from formalized religion (Mackay 2004). Their strong connection with "place and land" is consistent with a highly spiritual orientation (Bouma 2006).

Therefore, how one perceives the terms *religion* and *spirituality* is highly context and culture specific. For South Africans, the two are inextricably linked, while in Australia they are distinctly different terms that arouse different emotional responses and different levels of following. Hence, the question in the current study, asking respondents to rate their level of spiritual/religious happiness and meaning, was likely to generate different perceptions among participants from different countries. Given that nations also vary in the extent to which their people are homogeneous, particularly with respect to religion, then this point becomes even more pertinent.

Well-Being Across Profiles of Spiritual/Religious Happiness and Meaning

A second aim of the study was to examine the well-being of groups of individuals (clusters) sharing similar profiles of spiritual/religious happiness and meaning. Four clusters were generated as described in the results section (high, happiness, meaning, and low). When comparing the four clusters in terms of well-being (operationalized as satisfaction with life, general happiness rating, and general meaning rating), participants in the *High* cluster group were more satisfied with their lives and reported higher general meaning and happiness ratings than those in the other three clusters, although general happiness was highest among participants in both the *High* and *Happy* clusters. As expected, the low cluster was found to have the lowest level of meaning. Clearly, participants in the high and to a lesser extent in the happy cluster reported more substantial benefits in well-being. This is consistent with a considerable body of literature supporting the positive relationship between spirituality and well-being (e.g., see the meta-analysis by Chida et al. 2009).

When we examined clusters by country, the most striking finding was that the majority of South Africans (84.6%) were included in the *High* cluster (high spiritual happiness and meaning ratings) which is associated with the highest ratings on well-being. Interestingly, participants living in a context where religion represents a source of both happiness and meaningfulness, such as South Africa, but falling in the *Low* cluster (i.e., reporting low levels of spiritual/religious happiness and meaning) also reported lower levels of general meaning. To put it simply, it seems that a cultural context supporting religion and spirituality adversely impacts the well-being of those who do not share the same experiences as their fellow compatriots.

In support of these findings, Diener et al. (2011) found that religious people reported higher levels of well-being if they lived in a religious nation, particularly for nations experiencing difficult life conditions. Nonreligious people also fared well if they lived in a country that was also not highly religious. However, if individuals were not religious yet lived in a highly religious nation, then their well-being was likely to be negatively impacted. Similarly, if individuals were religious but lived in a nation that was not high on religion, their well-being was reduced. These authors suggested a "person-culture fit effect" underscoring the importance of social and cultural factors inherent within nations. However, causality cannot necessarily be assumed as other variables, such as socioeconomic factors, might also have played a role. For example, Rule (2007) showed that religiosity in South Africa is positively associated with material quality of life and self-assessed satisfaction with life. Participants from Portugal, though reporting their affiliation to a religion in the highest percentage within the study sample, were quite spread across the clusters, demonstrating varied perceived levels of spiritual/religious happiness and meaning and moderately high well-being. On the contrary in Australia, where ascribing to a religion is not so prevalent, the effects of being in the *Low* cluster did not turn out to be as detrimental to well-being (more specifically, general meaning) as they were to the South African sample. In fact, the Australian sample had the highest rating on satisfaction with life of all the countries, despite the low percentage of religious people. It may be that this lack of religion is compensated by the high level of spirituality presumed to be experienced by the Australian sample and by the perception that one is a good fit with their fellow citizens in terms of their religious outlook.

In most countries, high spiritual/religious happiness ratings by themselves (the *Happy* cluster) appeared to be more important for well-being evaluated in terms of satisfaction with life and general happiness, than were high spiritual/religious meaningfulness ratings by themselves (the *Meaning* cluster). This is an interesting point, as it suggests that a certain percentage of individuals (even though not very high across countries) perceive happiness with their spirituality but do not associate spirituality/religiousness with a similarly high level of meaning. Conversely, high levels of spiritual/religious meaning overall contribute to meaningfulness in general. These findings, confirmed by the analysis of the correlation between happiness and meaningfulness in the spiritual/religious domain, highlight the importance of distinguishing between hedonic and eudaemonic components of well-being, and more specifically between happiness and meaningfulness (Delle Fave et al. 2011b).

Study Limitations and Challenges for Future Research

The findings obtained in our study raise some issues to be taken into account in future research. First of all, if we accept that measures of spirituality conflate aspects of religion (Koenig 2008), and that culture is a significant influence on how spirituality is perceived (Bouma 2006), then the scales commonly used to measure spirituality may not be appropriate for and consistent across all countries and cultures. This point is most salient for countries like Australia, where the association between religion and spirituality are not strong, but may be less of an issue for countries such as South Africa where spirituality and religion are more closely intertwined. The diversity in how these key constructs are perceived makes cross-cultural comparisons very complex, but an understanding of these cultural variations enables more accurate interpretations. This is where the use of qualitative data as espoused by Delle Fave et al. (2011b) in the development of the EHHI can be highly informative and beneficial.

Secondly, the current study asked individuals to indicate their religious denomination. However, indicating affiliation to a religion and actually practicing in accordance with it can be two separate aspects, which were not distinguished in the current study. In future, more detail is needed about the nature and extent to which one is religious and spiritual so that less inferences are made by researchers about these dimensions.

Moreover, asking participants to rate their perceived levels of meaningfulness and happiness within the spiritual/religious domain can be a confusing task for some respondents, especially if the participants do not consider themselves as religious or spiritual. Further detail and clarification are needed in this regard.

Finally, there might be some cultural differences in tendency to give high ratings for socially desirable behaviors. For instance, overreporting of church attendance consistently appears in some North American countries but does not appear in the European surveys (Brenner 2011a). Although attendance is a biased measure of actual behavior, it may be a good indicator of religiosity. Brenner (2011b) also found that identity importance predicts overreported attendance. In cultures where religious identity is viewed as important, people will more often overreport religious service attendance.

It is also important to note that the sample only contains respondents aged between 30 and 50 years of age and only westernized countries. Moreover, only a small sample of the total population from each nation has been included in the current study, so it is difficult to ascertain how representative each sample is of the target population (each nation). More work is needed with more diverse samples to determine if the findings are more generalizable.

In sum, the findings from this study support previous literature indicating that there are distinct differences among countries in the extent to which people are religious and spiritual. The current study has also underscored the importance of using qualitative and quantitative methods to explore the relationship between well-being and religion/spirituality and has provided more refined detail about the cultural enablers and constraints which can affect this relationship.

References

Abdel-Khalek, A. M. (2006). Happiness, health, and religiosity: Significant relations. *Mental Health, Religion and Culture, 9*, 85–97.

Allport, G., & Ross, J. M. (1967). Personal religious orientation and prejudice. *Journal of Personality and Social Psychology, 5*, 432–443.

Ano, G. G., & Vasconcelles, E. B. (2005). Religious coping and psychological adjustment to stress: A meta-analysis. *Journal of Clinical Psychology, 61*, 461–480.

Bellingham, R., Cohen, B., Jones, T., & Spaniol, L. (1989). Connectedness: Some skills for spiritual health. *American Journal of Health Promotion, 4*, 18–31.

Bickel, C., Ciarrocchi, J., Sheers, N., Estdt, B., Powell, D., & Pargament, K. (1998). Perceived stress, religious coping styles, and depressive affect. *Journal of Psychology and Christianity, 17*, 33–42.

Bouma, G. (2006). *Australian soul: Religion and spirituality in the twenty-first century*. Port Melbourne: Cambridge University Press.

Brady, M. J., Peterman, A. H., Fitchett, G., Mo, M., & Cella, D. (1999). A case for including spirituality in quality of life measurement in oncology. *Psycho-Oncology, 8*, 417–428.

Brenner, P. S. (2011a). Exceptional behavior or exceptional identity? Overreporting of church attendance in the U.S. *Public Opinion Quarterly, 75*(1), 19–41.

Brenner, P. S. (2011b). Identity importance and the overreporting of religious service attendance: Multiple imputation of religious attendance using the American time use study and the general social survey. *Journal for the Scientific Study of Religion, 50*(1), 103–115.

Burnell, B. M., Beukes, R. B. I., & Esterhuyse, K. G. F. (2009). The relationship between spiritual well-being and a sense of meaning in life in late adolescence in South Africa. *Practical Theology in South Africa, 24*(1), 1–31.

Chida, Y., Steptoe, A., & Powell, L. H. (2009). Religiosity/spirituality and mortality. *Psychotherapy and Psychosomatics, 78*, 81–90.

Coppa, R., & Delle Fave, A. (2007). Pratica religiosa ed esperienza ottimale: una prospettiva eudaimonica. In A. Delle Fave (Ed.), *La condivisione del benessere. Il contributo della Psicologia Positiva* (pp. 73–93). Milano: Franco Angeli.

Coppa, R., & Delle Fave, A. (2009). Esperienza ottimale nella pratica religiosa e processo di attaccamento nella relazione con Dio. In G. Rossi & M. Aletti (Eds.), *Psicologia della religione e teoria dell'attaccamento* (pp. 95–106). Roma: Aracne Editrice.

Cummins, R. A., Eckersley, R., Lo, S. K., Davern, M., Hunter, B., & Okerstrom, E. (2004). The Australian unity wellbeing index: An overview. *Social Indicators Network News, 76*, 1–4.

Delle Fave, A., Massimini, F., & Bassi, M. (2011a). *Psychological selection and optimal experience across cultures*. Dordrecht: Springer.

Delle Fave, A., Brdar, I., Freire, T., Vella-Brodrick, D., & Wissing, M. P. (2011b). The eudaimonic and hedonic components of happiness: Qualitative and quantitative findings. *Social Indicators Research, 100*, 185–207. (Published online: 4 May 2010.)

Diener, E., Tay, L., & Myers, D. (2011). The religion paradox: If religion makes people happy, why are so many dropping out? *Journal of Personality and Social Psychology*. doi:10.1037/a0024402.

Eckersley, R. M. (2007). Culture, spirituality, religion and health: Looking at the big picture. *Medical Journal of Australia, 186*, S54–S56.

Emmons, R. A. (2005). Striving for the sacred: Personal goals, life meaning, and religion. *Journal of Social Issues, 61*, 731–745.

Emmons, R. A. (2006). Spirituality. In M. Csikszentmihalyi & I. Csikszentmihalyi (Eds.), *A life worth living. Contributions to positive psychology* (pp. 62–81). New York: Oxford University Press.

Emmons, R. A., & McCullough, M. E. (2004). *The psychology of gratitude*. New York: Oxford University Press.

Fahlberg, L. L., & Fahlberg, L. A. (1991). Exploring spirituality and consciousness with an expanded science: Beyond the ego with empiricism, phenomenology, and contemplation. *American Journal of Health Promotion, 5*, 273–281.

Fredrickson, B. L. (2002). How does religion benefit health and well-being? Are positive emotions active ingredients? *Psychological Inquiry, 13*(3), 209–213.

Geyer, A. L., & Baumeister, R. F. (2005). Religion, morality, and self-control. In R. F. Paloutzian & C. L. Park (Eds.), *Handbook of the psychology of religion and spirituality* (pp. 412–432). New York: The Guilford Press.

Gillum, R. F., & Ingram, D. D. (2006). Frequency of attendance at religious services, hypertension, and blood pressure: The Third National Health and Nutrition Examination Survey. *Psychosomatic Medicine, 68*, 382–385.

Howell, R. T., Kern, M. L., & Lyubomirsky, S. (2007). Health benefits: Meta-analytically determining the impact of well-being on objective health outcomes. *Health Psychology Review, 1*, 83–136.

Jenkins, R., & Pargament, K. (1995). Religion and spirituality as resources for coping with cancer. *Journal of Psychosocial Oncology, 13*, 51–74.

Joshanloo, M. (2010). Investigation of the contribution of spirituality and religiousness to hedonic and eudaimonic well-being in Iranian young adults. *Journal of Happiness Studies*. doi:10.1007/s10902-010-9236-4.

King, M., Speck, P., & Thomas, A. (1995). The royal free interview for religious and spiritual beliefs: Development and standardization. *Psychological Medicine, 25*, 1125–1134.

King, M., Speck, P., & Thomas, A. (2001). The royal free interview for religious and spiritual beliefs: Development and validation of a self-report version. *Psychological Medicine, 31*, 1015–1023.

Koenig, H. G. (2008). Concerns about measuring 'spirituality' in research. *The Journal of Nervous and Mental Disease, 196*, 349–355.

Koenig, H. G., McCullough, M., & Larson, D. B. (2001). *Handbook of religion and health*. New York: Oxford University Press.

Larson, D. B., Koenig, H. G., Kaplan, B. H., Greenberg, R. S., Logue, E., & Taylor, H. A. (1989). The impact of religion on men's blood pressure. *Journal of Religion and Health, 28*, 265–278.

Mackay, H. (2004). *Right and wrong: How to decide for yourself*. Sydney: Hodder.

Massimini, F., & Delle Fave, A. (1991). Religion and cultural evolution. *Zygon, 1*, 27–47.

McClain, C. S., Rosenfeld, B., & Breitbart, W. (2003). Effect of spiritual well-being on end-of-life despair in terminally-ill cancer patients. *Lancet, 361*, 1603–1607.

McCullough, M. E., Pargament, K. I., & Thoresen, C. E. (2000). *Forgiveness: Theory, research, and practice*. New York: The Guilford Press.

Myers, D. G. (2000). The funds, friends and faith of happy people. *American Psychologist, 55*, 56–67.

Mytko, J. J., & Knight, S. J. (1999). Body, mind and spirit: Towards the integration of religiosity and spirituality in cancer quality of life research. *Psycho-Oncology, 8*, 439–450.

NationMaster. (2010). *Nations of the world*. www.nationmaster.com/country. Downloaded 12 Sept 2011.

O'Collins, G., & Farrugia, E. G. (1991). *A concise dictionary of theology*. New York: Paulist Press.

Paloutzian, R. F., & Park, C. L. (Eds.). (2005). *Handbook of the psychology of religion and spirituality*. New York: The Guilford Press.

Park, C. (2005). Religion as a meaning-making framework in coping with life stress. *Journal of Social Issues, 61*, 707–729.

Patel, C. J., Ramgoon, S., & Paruk, Z. (2009). Exploring religion, race and gender as factors in the life satisfaction and religiosity of young South African adults. *South African Journal of Psychology, 39*(3), 266–274.

Peach, H. G. (2003). Religion, spirituality and health: How should Australia's medical professionals respond? *Medical Journal of Australia, 178*, 86–88.

Rule, S. (2007). Religiosity and quality of life in South Africa. *Social Indicators Research, 81*, 417–434.

Sedikides, C. (2010). Why does religiosity persist? *Personality and Social Psychology Review, 14*, 3–6.

Shahabi, L., Powell, L. H., Musick, M. A., Pargament, K. I., Thoresen, C. E., Williams, D., Underwood, L., & Ory, M. A. (2002). Correlates of self-perceptions of spirituality in American adults. *Annals of Behavioral Medicine, 24*, 59–68.

Snoep, L. (2008). Religiousness and happiness in three nations: A research note. *Journal of Happiness Studies, 9*, 207–211.

Sperry, K., & Shafranske, E. P. (Eds.). (2005). *Spiritually oriented psychotherapy*. Washington, DC: American Psychological Association.

Spiegel, D., & Fawzy, I. F. (2002). Psychosocial interventions and prognosis in cancer. In H. G. Koenig & H. J. Cohen (Eds.), *The link between religion and health. Psychoneuroimmunology and the faith factor* (pp. 84–100). New York: Oxford University Press.

Suhail, K., & Chaudry, H. R. (2004). Predictors of subjective well-being in an eastern Muslim culture. *Journal of Social and Clinical Psychology, 23*, 359–376.

Tarakeshwar, N., Stanton, J., & Pargament, K. J. (2003). Religion. An overlooked dimension in cross-cultural psychology. *Journal of Cross-Cultural Psychology, 34*, 377–394.

The Association of Religion Data Archives. (2009). www.thearda.com. Downloaded 14 Sept. 2011.

Tiliouine, H. (2009). Measuring satisfaction with religiosity and its contribution to the personal well-being index in a Muslim sample. *Applied Research in Quality of Life, 4*, 91–108.

Tsuang, M. T., & Simpson, J. C. (2008). Commentary on Koenig (2008). Concerns about measuring 'spirituality' in research. *The Journal of Nervous and Mental Disease, 196*, 647–649.

Tsuang, M. T., Simpson, J. C., Koenen, K. C., Kremen, W. S., & Lyons, M. J. (2007). Spiritual well-being and health. *The Journal of Nervous and Mental Disease, 195*, 673–680.

Van Dierendonck, D. (2011). Spirituality as an essential determinant for the Good Life, its importance relative to self-determinant psychological needs. *Journal of Happiness Studies*. doi:10.1007/s10902-011-9286-2.

Vaughan, F. (1991). Spiritual issues in psychotherapy. *Journal of Transpersonal Psychology, 23*, 105–119.

Walsh, K., King, M., Jones, L., Tookman, A., & Blizard, R. (2002). Spiritual beliefs may affect outcome of bereavement: Prospective study. *British Medical Journal, 324*, 1551–1555.

WHOQOL Group. (2006). A cross-cultural study of spirituality, religion, and personal beliefs as components of quality of life. *Social Science & Medicine, 62*, 1486–1497.

Wills, E. (2009). Spirituality and subjective well-being: Evidences for a new domain in the Personal Well-Being Index. *Journal of Happiness Studies, 10*, 49–69.

Zaccagnini, J. L., Delle Fave, A., & Sanabria, E. (2010, June 23–26). *Religious practice and optimal experience in a Spanish Catholic sample*. Presentation at the 5th European conference on positive psychology, Copenhagen.

Zinnbauer, B. J., & Pargament, K. I. (2005). Religiousness and spirituality. In R. F. Paloutzian & C. L. Park (Eds.), *Handbook of the psychology of religion and spirituality* (pp. 21–42). New York: The Guilford Press.

Chapter 9
The Relationship of South African Consumers' Living Standards and Demographic Variables with Their Life Satisfaction

Leona Ungerer

Introduction

People are bombarded daily with powerful messages that the good life is 'the goods life' (Kasser 2004). Advertisements, for instance, often imply that happiness and well-being come from attaining wealth and from the purchase and acquisition of goods and services. People may consequently believe that they need and want certain products and service to enhance their well-being (Csikszentmihaly, in Schmuck and Sheldon 2001).

Furthermore, materialism has been singled out as the dominant consumer ideology in modern consumer behaviour (Cross 2004). This construct refers to the importance ascribed to the ownership and acquisition of material goods in achieving major life goals or desired states (Richins and Dawson, in Richins 2004, p. 210). According to Richins and Dawson (in Richins 2004), material values include three domains: the use of possessions to judge a person's own success and those of others, how central possessions are in a person's life, and how strongly a person believes that possessions and their acquisition will lead to his or her happiness and life satisfaction.

The above may also apply to South Africa. According to Goosen and Rossouw (2006), an unprecedented wave of violent crime and the constant stimulation of a consumer culture are directly related in South Africa. Media and marketing vehemently expose thousands of people who are excluded from the economy to an exaltation of a mobile, urbanised consumer which most of them will never be. This constant stimulation of people's desires results in a state of desire wear-out, which manifests in depression, burnout, feelings of meaninglessness and a chronic desire for the next 'high' or the most recent innovation. This crisis especially manifests amongst members of the black middle class, who have been swiftly catapulted from apartheid's suppressed

L. Ungerer (✉)
University of South Africa, Pretoria, South Africa
e-mail: Ungerlm@unisa.ac.za

H.H. Knoop and A. Delle Fave (eds.), *Well-Being and Cultures: Perspectives from Positive Psychology*, Cross-Cultural Advancements in Positive Psychology 3, DOI 10.1007/978-94-007-4611-4_9, © Springer Science+Business Media Dordrecht 2013

desires to post-apartheid's absolutised desires. Furthermore, they believe that it is not surprising that thousands of people from desperate poverty resort to violence and crime, driven by an overstimulated but chronic desire for 'the good life'.

Another factor that may contribute to the above is the inequality in the distribution of wealth in South Africa, as reflected in one of the highest Gini- coefficients in the world (0.67 in 2010) (http://www.popai.co.za/gini-coefficient-amongst-highest/). (A Gini coefficient of '1' is an indication of complete income inequality with one person having all the income, whereas a Gini coefficient of '0' is indicative of complete equality with everybody earning an equal income). Van Aardt (in Shevel and Klein 2008) referred to South Africa's unequal wealth distribution as a 'recipe for disaster'. He pointed out that, although there has been a significant increase in the wealth of black consumers, nearly 22.5 million South Africans live at the breadline or below it. Furthermore, Jammine (in Shevel and Klein 2008) indicated that there are currently many more members of the black middle class, but there are relatively few black people who are extremely wealthy in South Africa.

Events such as the above explain why Sirgy and Lee (2008) pointed out that dramatic changes in society have created opportunities to develop and expand market research beyond product and service satisfaction – the traditional focus of the marketing discipline – to also focus on consumers' life satisfaction. Sirgy and Lee (2008) believe that marketing paradigms have evolved to culminate in well-being marketing. It is a business philosophy that guides managers to develop and implement marketing strategies that focus on enhancing consumer well-being throughout the consumer/product life cycle and to do so safely in relation to consumers, other publics and the environment (Sirgy and Lee 2008, p. 378).

Sirgy and Lee (2008, p. 378) define consumer well-being as a desired state of objective and subjective well-being, which is involved in the various stages of the consumer/product life cycle in relation to consumer goods. Well-being consequently is an essential concept in understanding the 'whole person' and is a key influence on how people respond to marketing messages. It is an increasing area of concern for Western governments and is entering the economic and marketing literature (Higgs 2003).

Developments such as the above have culminated in the recent establishment of the field of transformative consumer research. Transformative consumer research is a dynamic and evolving paradigm, and its normative goal is to improve well-being – a state of flourishing that involves health, happiness and prosperity. Mick et al. (2011) identify a number of changes in society which necessitate consumer research that closely focuses on well-being. Amongst these are the influence of consumption on the global natural environment, severe economic imbalances which lead to political and social tensions that are threatening peace and security, mounting household debt and addictions to various consumer products and activities experienced by millions of people.

Mick et al. (2011) point out that the answer to the question of what the good life is partly lies in people's personal and collective consumption behaviours. Both the Worldwatch Institute and the Commission on the Measurement of Economic Performance and Social Progress argue that the nature and extent of the 'good life' can no longer be mainly judged according to a criterion of wealth or gross domestic product. Instead, the predominant standard must shift to well-being, and well-being has become fundamentally and intricately joined with the acquiring, consuming and disposing of goods and services.

The issue of 'what makes a good life', however, is fraught with cultural assumptions (Wierzbicka 2009). Societies and individuals, for instance, differ in the degree to which they believe that life satisfaction is a key attribute of the good life (Diener and Suh 1997). Most subjective well-being research, however, has been undertaken in Western countries. Kitayama and Markus (2000) suggested that most well-being research is based on middle-class American meanings and practices. According to Diener and Suh (2000), very poor countries such as those in Africa, are still under-represented in research on subjective well-being. Al-Wugayan and Suprenant (2006) further referred to a growing concern that most existing knowledge about consumer behaviour has been derived from research undertaken in America and a few Western European nations, comprising less than 6% of the world population. An aim of the current study was therefore to make a contribution in this regard by yielding data in the South African context.

The life satisfaction of the broad South African population was investigated in a number of studies such as those by Neff (2007). These studies were based on a social indicator approach – information about people's well-being was used to guide public policy. These subjective social indicators supplement measures of the objective standard of living (Schwarz and Strack 1999).

Probably the most in-depth investigation of South African consumers' subjective well-being is that of Higgs (2007). He developed a comprehensive model of consumers' subjective well-being, which he termed the Everyday Quality of Life Index (EQLi). He believes that the vision of improving service delivery in South Africa makes the measurement of people's quality of life in SA a greater imperative than before. His model provides a measurement framework that has shown stability over time and enables progress towards a better life for all to be quantitatively measured. His model includes factors such as socio-economic status, urbanisation, health, stress/pressure, quality of the environment, satisfaction of human needs, connectivity, optimism, subjective well-being and overall well-being. He based his model on data obtained in nationally representative samples during a number of consumer surveys undertaken by a well-known South African market research organisation.

This study builds on existing research on South African consumers' subjective well-being by focusing solely on the life satisfaction of South African household purchase decision-makers. These consumers play a pivotal role in household decision-making, and therefore the consumer domain, as will be evident below.

Higgs (2008) pointed out that South Africa is ideally suited to market research because of its cultural diversity and its high Gini coefficient. A marketplace as diverse as in South Africa, composed of many different people, with different backgrounds, interests, needs and wants, especially lends itself to market segmentation – the practice of dividing a market into smaller specific segments sharing similar characteristics (Tranter et al. 2009, p. 42).

The purpose for segmenting a market is to enable a company to focus its marketing programme on the subset of consumers that are most likely to purchase its products and services. A further point to consider is, given the characteristics of the company's products and services, what type of decision-maker will most likely be interested in purchasing them (http://www.businessplans.org-/Segment.html). Marketers are particularly interested in the demographic and media profiles of the household decision-makers. Although they are not necessarily the household decision-makers for all products, the current research is based on data obtained from consumers who are responsible for their households' purchases.

In light of the above, it may be important to investigate whether increases in material prosperity will be accompanied by increases in life satisfaction amongst purchase decision-makers in South Africa, with its high degree of cultural diversity and its high Gini coefficient. A tool which would be useful in investigating this relationship is the Living Standards Measure (LSM). The LSM, developed by the South African Advertising Research Foundation (SAARF), is one of the most widely used marketing segmentation tools in South Africa. The LSM is a wealth measure, based on standard of living (http://www.saarf.co.za). The latest LSM segmentation approach classifies households into ten distinct LSM groupings, based on their access to services and durables, and geographic indicators as determinants of their standard of living. Ethnic group is not considered as a segmentation variable in the LSM.

Subjective Well-Being

Diener (in Schimmack 2008) originally proposed that subjective well-being has three distinct components: life satisfaction, positive affect and negative affect. More recently, Diener, Suh, Lucas, and Smith (in Schimmack 2008) also included satisfaction in specific live domains (domain satisfaction, for instance, satisfaction with health) in the definition of subjective well-being.

Researchers often distinguish between cognitive and affective components of subjective well-being. Life satisfaction and domain satisfaction are considered cognitive components because they are based on evaluative beliefs (attitudes) about one's life. In contrast, positive affect and negative affect assess the affective component of subjective well-being and reflect the amount of pleasant and unpleasant feelings people experience in their lives. Life satisfaction has been identified as a distinct construct representing a cognitive and global evaluation of the quality of one's life as a whole (Pavot and Diener 1993). Although life satisfaction is correlated with the affective components of subjective well-being, it forms a separate factor from the other types of well-being (Lucas, Diener and Suh, in Pavot and Diener 2008).

Subjective well-being is an overarching domain that includes a broad collection of constructs that relate to individuals' subjective evaluation of the quality of their lives (Lucas 2008). A comprehensive assessment of subjective well-being therefore requires separate measures of both life satisfaction and the affective components of subjective well-being (Diener and Seligman, in Pavot and Diener 2008).

There is currently no single conceptual scheme that unites the entire field of subjective well-being in terms of its determinants. Both bottom-up and top-down influences may impact on peoples' subjective well-being. Top-down influences refer to broad personality and cognitive factors that influence subjective well-being, while bottom-up influences refer to events and circumstances, including external events, situations and demographics that can influence subjective well-being (Diener et al. 2003).

The Relationship Between People's Demographic Variables and Their Life Satisfaction

The relationship between people's demographic characteristics and their satisfaction with life has been investigated extensively. According to Diener and Lucas (1999), demographic factors such as people's health, income, educational background and marital status account for only a small amount of the variance in well-being measures. This is partially due to the fact that the effects of demographic variables are probably mediated by psychological processes such as people's goals and coping abilities.

The relationship between purchase decision-makers' satisfaction with life and some of their demographic characteristics, however, had to be confirmed in this research because a person's demographic profile may influence his or her subjective well-being to some degree, which means that demographic data can potentially add to the overall understanding of the person's subjective experience (Pavot and Diener 2004). Furthermore, these characteristics are often used as segmentation bases, or combined with other segmentation bases, which may point to the need to investigate their relationship with purchase decision-makers' life satisfaction.

Age and Life Satisfaction

Although a small decline in life satisfaction is occasionally found with age, the relation is eliminated when other variables such as income are controlled (Shmotkin, in Diener et al. 1999). In other studies, it was found that life satisfaction often increases, or at least does not drop with age (Horley and Lavery, in Diener et al. 1999; Stock, Okun, Haring and Witter, in Diener et al. 1999). In several studies, there was little difference in terms of subjective well-being between black and white older people (Argyle 1999), although people from various ethnic groups tend to differ in terms of life satisfaction earlier in their lives.

Gender and Life Satisfaction

La Barbera and Gurhan (1997) pointed out that no significant gender differences in subjective well-being were found in several classic studies. In those studies where significant gender differences in subjective well-being are indeed found, definitive answers regarding the causes of these differences are seldom provided. Nolen-Hoeksema and Rusting (in Lucas and Gohm 2000) reviewed a number of possible mechanisms for these differences and conclude that personality explanations and social context explanations are most promising. They conclude that the issue whether gender differences in subjective well-being exist cannot be answered with a simple yes or no. It depends on the component of subjective well-being which is measured and the way these components are measured. In light of the fact that gender as such appears to have marginal significance in predicting subjective well-being, La Barbera and Gurhan (1997) suggested that people's gender and their perceived gender roles, for instance, should rather be investigated in subjective well-being research.

Ethnic Group and Life Satisfaction

International surveys of life satisfaction have shown that nations differ from each other in terms of life satisfaction and that ethnic groups within nations differ from each other too (Diener et al. 2003). Argyle (1999) quoted research by Møller, done in South Africa and published in 1989, in which it was found that white South Africans were happiest, followed by Indians, coloureds and blacks. Møller (2007), however, pointed out that black South Africans' improved living standards under democracy resulted in an increase in their life satisfaction. She points out that their satisfaction with life increased drastically after the first democratic elections, but this trend faded rapidly and in later surveys blacks scored significantly lower than other South Africans on satisfaction with life. An explanation she offers is that their material aspirations have not been met. All in all, Kingdon and Knight (in O'Leary 2007) indicated that South Africans' life satisfaction is not related to their ethnic group as such; it is rather related to their varying circumstances.

Veenhoven and his colleagues (in Argyle 1999) postulated that ethnic minorities' lower happiness, as identified in some studies, are mainly due to their lower incomes, education and job status. When these variables are controlled, the effect of ethnicity is reduced, and in some studies removed completely. Taking this into consideration, it was attempted in this research to control for purchase decision-makers' income to test whether the differences between the various ethnic groups would be still evident if this is the case.

Income and Life Satisfaction

Already in 1995, Oropesa (1995) pointed out that the relationship between people's material quality of life and their subjective quality of life in modern developed societies is often debated. A consistent finding is that people's objective conditions often correlate only weakly with their subjective well-being (Diener and Fujita 1995; Christoph 2010). This may be because people tend to adapt over time to their conditions, which lessens the impact of their external circumstances on their well-being.

Furthermore, people's expectations are important determinants of their subjective well-being (Triandis 2000). According to Michalos' (in Christoph 2010) Multiple Discrepancies Theory, people compare what they actually have with (a) their personal aspirations, (b) the situation of relevant others, (c) what they deserve, (d) their basic needs and (e) intertemporal comparisons as contrasting their current situation with the past, with their past expectations about today or the expectations they have for the future.

A further consistent finding on this relationship is that people's income correlates with their well-being, both within and across countries (Diener, Diener and Diener, in Diener and Fujita 1995), and that the relation between financial satisfaction and life satisfaction is stronger in developing countries (Diener and Diener in Diener and Fujita 1995). However, more recently it became evident that the weak relationship between people's material situation and their subjective well-being may partly be explained by the insufficiencies of income as an indicator for people's material situation. Alternative measures for people's material situation, particularly wealth measures, reveal a stronger relationship between people's material well-being and their subjective well-being (Christoph 2010).

Christoph (2010) pointed out that the positive correlation between income and subjective well-being at the individual level is rather low, especially when contrasted to the one found in aggregate data. It furthermore is much stronger for people in the lower income brackets than for those with higher incomes and is curvilinear. Although there appears to be general agreement that there is a connection between income and subjective well-being, the theoretical foundations of this relationship are not clear.

According to Argyle (in Christoph 2010), income measures and measures of subjective well-being could be expected to correlate positively because having more money offers opportunities such as a higher standard of living and better housing. Christoph (2010) identifies at least four different theoretical approaches in the literature on well-being that aim to explain the link between income and well-being: (1) need theory or livability theory, (2) the relative standards model, (3) the cultural approach and (4) specific variants of set-point theory like Cummins' (in Christoph 2010) 'Homeostatic Theory of Subjective Well-being'.

In summary, the relationship between people's income and their life satisfaction has been investigated extensively in previous research, and a number of theories have been developed to explain the relationship between these two variables. According to Cummins (2000), there appears not to be a strong causal link between people's income and their subjective well-being, and more complex models are probably required to explain the relationship between these two constructs.

It has been found in international studies that people's well-being correlates with their wealth up to a point where greater wealth yields considerable improvements in people's feelings of well-being. But, beyond that point, additional wealth has little incremental effect on subjective well-being (Higgs 2007). Higgs (2007) pointed out that there is a point where increasing income does not produce any increase in well-being (as measured by the four components that he identified in his research, namely, the cognitive component, two affective components and what he refers to as a striving component). For South Africa, this point occurred at an income of about R8,000. He based this finding on an omnibus survey in July 2002, which covered the major metropolitan areas of South Africa, included adults over the age of 18 years and was stratified by ethnic group, gender, language and formal/informal housing type. The total sample size was 2,000.

Higgs (2007) pointed out that he found that happiness and quality of life measures flatten out at monthly household incomes of R3,000 for health, R6,500 for happiness and R11,500 for overall quality of life. He points out, however, that self-reported income data in South Africa are extremely unreliable. Furthermore, the minimum income needed to survive, or to attain a reasonable quality of life, depends on where a person lives (in terms of product purchasing parity), the size of his or her family, other dependants, for instance, the extended family in black cultures and other monetary assets. He bases these findings on a metropolitan area survey of 2,000 South African adults in winter 2002, summer 2003 and a national study in all areas of 3,500 adults in winter 2003.

Research Problem

The research problem investigated in this research study was whether there are differences amongst purchase decision-makers in various LSM super groups' life satisfaction. In order to investigate the problem, the following research questions are relevant: What is the nature of the relationships between the living standards of purchase decision-makers and their life satisfaction?

The primary purpose of this research was to investigate to what extent life satisfaction, as measured by Diener et al. (1985) Satisfaction with Life Scale (SWLS), differs across the LSM groupings that are used within a multicultural South African context and to investigate the nature of the relationships between these constructs.

Therefore, the general aim was to investigate whether there is relationship between the life satisfaction of purchase decision-makers and their living standards. The empirical aims for this research are to determine whether life satisfaction vary for purchase decision-makers across different LSM super groups and to investigate the relationship between purchase decision-makers' LSM level and their life satisfaction.

Method

Participants

The sample consisted of 2,566 household purchase decision-makers of whom 57.5% were males and 42.5% were females. The average age of the respondents was 40.41 years (SD = 15.14 years). More than half of the respondents (55.80%) were in relationships where they shared a household. In terms of being purchase decision-makers (PDMs), this group of respondents would most probably be responsible for the purchases for their households, whereas the remainder of the sample might typically only shop for themselves. The majority of the sample (68.28%) had an African language as their home language, whereas 17.07% were Afrikaans-speaking and 14.65% were English-speaking. Only 28.8% of the respondents had completed matric or a higher educational level. Similarly, only 46.4% of the respondents were employed full-time or part-time. The household income data of only 2,156 respondents were obtained because some refused to provide this information. Of those who responded, 25% had a monthly household income of less than R900 per month, 37% had an income of between R900 and R2,999, whereas 38% earned more than R3,000 per month. In terms of South Africa's main ethnic groups, the sample consisted mainly of black people (69%), whereas 16% were white, 11% were coloured and 4% were Indian.

Nearly 60% of the sample lived in metropolitan areas. This fact may have important implications for this research because marketers have found differences in consumer purchasing patterns amongst urban, suburban and rural areas (Schiffman and Kanuk 2007). Consumers' degree of urbanisation is therefore an important segmentation variable that influences what products are distributed, how they are distributed and how they are priced and promoted (Arnould et al. 2004). The degree of urbanisation is also an important descriptor in the current research because people from the lower LSM groups tend to be found in rural areas, while those in higher LSM groups tend to reside in urban areas.

Four LSM super groups were subsequently created to investigate differences amongst them on life satisfaction. The LSM super groups were represented as follows in the sample: 33% was from LSM super group 1, 26% represented LSM super group 2, 16% represented LSM super group 3 and 24% was from LSM super group 4.

Since it is well known that ethnic groups may exhibit response patterns that bias results, and since the ethnic group variable tended to be strongly associated with the LSM super group variable, it was essential to determine to what extent respondents' ethnic group and their LSM grouping were related. More than 95% of purchase decision-makers in LSM super group 1 were black; within LSM super group 2, this percentage was almost 90%; in LSM super group 3, it was 67%; whereas only 11.6% of purchase decision-makers in LSM super group 4 were black. Ignoring the effect of purchase decision-makers' ethnic group would therefore be a serious threat to the validity of the findings because the respondents' ethnic group and their LSM grouping were strongly related.

Measuring Instruments

The Satisfaction with Life Scale

According to Tucker et al. (2006), people differ dramatically in what they require for a satisfying life, such as personal freedom, good health or a comfortable income. In light of the fact that the sources of life satisfaction vary widely amongst individuals, it can be expected to also vary across cultures and subcultures, gender and age groups and people living in prosperous countries compared to those living in developing countries.

The SWLS, a five-item scale developed by Diener et al. (1985), was used to measure the life satisfaction of consumers in this study. People's degree of life satisfaction is measured on a cognitive-judgemental level (Wissing and Van Eeden 2002) – they evaluate their life satisfaction subjectively by examining their life as a whole when responding to the SWLS. Respondents may use whatever sources they choose for evaluating how satisfied they are with their lives overall. Researchers are then able to compare groups, using items that are apparently free from culturally specific definitions, as well as from individuals' varying criteria for life satisfaction (Pavot and Diener, in Tucker et al. 2006). The main rationale for using this scale was the brevity of the scale, which is desirable in a large survey comprising several variables (Pavot and Diener 1993). The use of brief scales in surveys in emerging societies such as South Africa is strongly recommended (Burgess 2002).

Møller (2007) pointed out that a person's satisfaction with his/her life as a whole is one of the most widely used measures of subjective well-being internationally. The SWLS was judged to be a valid and reliable scale for measuring life satisfaction by Pavot and Diener (1993) and several others, such as Oishi (2000). The SWLS has demonstrated its reliability and validity amongst Korean (Suh, in Oishi 2000), mainland Chinese (Shao, in Oishi 2000) and Russian samples (Balatsky and Diener, in Oishi 2000). In these studies, the obtained Cronbach's alphas ranged from 0.41 to 0.94, with a mean of 0.78 (SD = 0.09).

Diener et al. (in Pavot and Diener 1993) conducted a principal-axis factor analysis on the SWLS, from which a single factor emerged, accounting for 66% of the variance of the scale. This single-factor solution has since been replicated (Arrindell, Meeuwesen and Huyse, in Pavot and Diener 1993; Blais, Vallerand, Pelletier and Briere, in Pavot and Diener 1993; Pavot, Diener, Colvin and Sandvik, in Pavot and Diener 1993). The consistent factor pattern across samples was found despite the fact that translations of the SWLS into French and Dutch, as well as the original version, were used. The SWLS therefore appears to measure a single dimension.

Pavot and Diener (1993), however, pointed out that the true meaning of high life satisfaction will not be fully understood before the cognitive processes involved in arriving at life satisfaction judgements have been determined. A crucial aspect in developing the construct validity of the SWLS will consequently be to understand the processes involved in arriving at a life satisfaction judgement.

However, a contentious issue in cross-cultural research is always whether measures developed in Western nations are valid in non-Western cultures. Diener (2000) found the SWLS to be valid and reliable for various cultural groups, whereas in South Africa, Wissing, Thekiso, Stapelberg, Van Quickelberge, Chaobi, Moroeng and Nienaber (in Wissing and Van Eeden 2002) found that the SWLS was reliable and valid for a Setswana-speaking group. Therefore, there was adequate support for the use of the scale within the culturally diverse sample targeted in this study.

In the original SWLS, respondents were required to indicate how strongly they agreed with the items on a seven-point Likert scale. However, I decided to adapt the response scale of the SWLS to a five-point scale because the broad South African population probably relates better to simplified response categories, compared to the original sample of college students which Diener et al. (1985) used when developing the SWLS. The response categories ranged from 1 (strongly disagree) to 5 (strongly agree). Despite this change, the reliability and validity corresponded to that of the original SWLS, corresponding with Pavot's (2008) observation that the SWLS is useful for the assessment of people across a wide range of educational levels and ages.

The LSM Measure

In this study, the new SAARF Universal LSM® scale that consists of 29 variables was used to determine in which of the ten LSM classifications the respondents fall. To reduce sampling variability to obtain groups of similar sizes, four LSM super groups were formed.

In deciding which groups to combine for further analyses, general market practice was taken into consideration, and the following super groups were created: LSM super group 1 (purchase decision-makers from LSM 1–3), LSM super group 2 (purchase decision-makers from LSM 4–5), LSM super group 3 (purchase decision-makers from LSM 6–7) and LSM super group 4 (purchase decision-makers from LSM 8–10).

Procedure

Four LSM super groups were created to investigate differences amongst them in terms of their life satisfaction. Data were obtained from consumers who were wholly, mainly or partly responsible for the day-to-day purchases of the household. The sample therefore consisted of adult South African purchase decision-makers.

Research Design

A quantitative research design, using a cross-sectional survey, was employed. The population for this research was defined as South African adults (16 years and older) that are primary consumers of fast-moving consumer goods. A stratified probability sample of 3,500 adults was selected for data collection purposes. The primary stratification variable was geographical region, using the nine provinces as a basis. The second stratification variable was community size, with included cities, large towns, small towns, villages and rural areas. The metro sample was a stratified probability sample consisting of 2,000 adults living in metropolitan areas. The non-metro sample also consisted of a stratified probability sample of 1,500 adults, but living in non-metropolitan areas. This sampling process resulted in 3,500 face-to-face, in-house interviews being undertaken with respondents in both metro and non-metropolitan areas. The research questionnaire included a screening question requiring respondents to indicate whether they were mainly responsible for purchasing fast-moving consumer goods for their households. This exclusion criterion resulted in a final sample of 2,566 adult South African household purchase decision-makers being suitable for analysis in this study.

Data Collection

The original English questionnaire was translated into isiZulu, isiXhosa, Setswana, Sesotho, Sepedi, and Afrikaans. In order to ensure that all translations were accurate, all questionnaires were back-translated to English and controlled for accuracy, in line with methods recommended by Van de Vijver and Leung (1997). Interviews were conducted in the language according to the preference of the respondent. All interviewers had a Senior Certificate qualification and were trained and thoroughly briefed before they conducted any interviews. The interviewers were representative of the South African society. All black interviewers were required to be proficient in four languages, whereas white, coloured and Indian interviewers were required to have command over at least two languages. Although all interviews were conducted under the constant supervision of trained and experienced supervisors, a minimum of 20% back-checking on each interviewer's work was conducted to ensure accuracy and consistency in terms of South Africa's main ethnic groups to prevent falsification of information and to verify sampling accuracy.

Results

The psychometric properties of the SWLS were established as a first step. The reliability of the SWLS was established by means of Cronbach's alpha and item-total correlations (see Table 9.1).

Table 9.1 Item analysis of the SWLS

Item	Corrected item-total correlation	Cronbach's alpha if item is deleted
All items		0.83
swl01	0.56	0.81
swl02	0.71	0.77
swl03	0.72	0.76
swl04	0.65	0.78
swl05	0.48	0.83

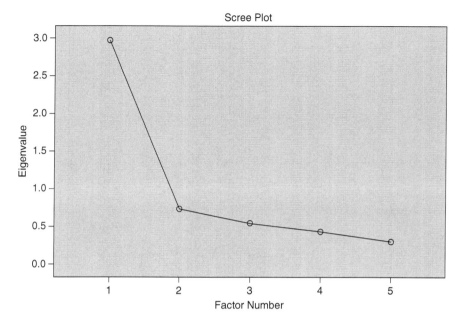

Fig. 9.1 Scree plot for exploratory factor analysis of the SWLS

The overall scale has an alpha value of 0.83. It is evident that scores on every item correlated highly with total test scores, but the last item ('If I could live my life over, I would change very little') was the weakest in terms of its convergence with other items. The reason may be that it mainly refers to the past, as pointed out by Pavot and Diener (1993). The above results confirm Oishi's (2000) observation that the SWLS has adequate reliability.

Validity of the SWLS

The factor structure of the SWLS was assessed by means of an exploratory factor analysis. It is clear that the scree plot shown in Fig. 9.1 supports the existence of a single factor. In addition, only one factor should be extracted when using the criterion of *eigenvalues* larger than 1.

Table 9.2 presents the obtained factor loadings. As was the case with the item-total correlations, item 5 was the weakest item due to its low factor loading. The remaining four items loaded relatively highly on the single factor (as reflected by values of above 0.6).

The findings above serve as a confirmation of the usefulness of the five-point response scale (as opposed to using the original seven-point scale) in this study, as well as in future research. It further appears that life satisfaction may be a meaningful

Table 9.2 Single-factor solution for SWLS

	Factor 1
swl01	0.624
swl02	0.813
swl03	0.822
swl04	0.722
swl05	0.518

and useful psychological construct. The SWLS items appear to hold together in a unified factor, suggesting that there is coherence to this measurement of life satisfaction (Pavot and Diener 1993). According to them, life satisfaction often forms a factor separate from affective indices of well-being. One of the reasons for this is that persons' conscious evaluation of their life circumstances may reflect conscious values and goals.

Differences Between Groups on Satisfaction with Life

Purchase decision-makers' satisfaction with life will firstly be investigated in terms of their demographic variables such as gender, age, ethnic group, income and the size of the community in which they live. It will then be investigated in terms of the LSM super groups created in this research.

Gender Effects on Satisfaction with Life

In order to determine whether there were significant differences amongst male and female purchase decision-makers in terms of their life satisfaction, a t test for independent means, was performed. The p-value of 0.151 [$t(2,564)=-1.43$] indicates that male and female purchase decision-makers did not differ significantly in terms of their life satisfaction.

Age Effects on Satisfaction with Life

The correlation between purchase decision-makers' age and their life satisfaction was statistically significant [$r(2,497)=0.09$, $p<0.001$]. This relationship indicates that the older purchase decision-makers were, the more satisfied they were with life. This correlation, however, is quite small and may consequently have little practical significance.

Table 9.3 Post hoc comparisons for differences between ethnic groups on life satisfaction

Cluster	N	1	2	3
		Subsets		
Black	1,769	3.02		
Coloured	282		3.33	
White	408			3.67
Indian	107			3.77

The Effect of Purchase Decision-Makers' Ethnic Group on Their Satisfaction with Life

Purchase decision-makers from different ethnic groups were also compared in terms of their satisfaction with life scores by means of an F test. There were statistically significant differences amongst purchase decision-makers in terms of their satisfaction with life, based on their ethnic group [$F(3)=78.8, p<0.001$]. A *partial eta* was calculated for the ANOVA to determine the effect size of this relationship. A value of 0.086 was found which, according to Pallant and Pallant (2007), represents a medium effect. Although significant, the effect size of this relationship was weak, as indicated by *partial eta-squared* equal to 0.11.

Table 9.3 presents the homogeneous subsets as created by Duncan's multiple comparison procedure, as well as the means for groups in each homogeneous subset resulting from the post hoc test which was undertaken in order to determine between which of the ethnic groups significant differences existed.

It is evident from a review of the subsets and the means for groups in each homogeneous subset in Table 9.3 that black purchase decision-makers were least satisfied with their lives, followed by coloured purchase decision-makers. White and Indian purchase decision-makers, who did not differ significantly in terms of their life satisfaction scores, were most satisfied with their lives.

In light of Veenhoven and his colleagues' (in Argyle 1999) suggestion that the effect of ethnicity on life satisfaction is reduced when income, education and job status are controlled, it was attempted in this research study to control for purchase decision-makers' income to test whether the differences between the various ethnic groups would be still evident if this is the case. A two-way analysis of variance was performed and the results are provided in Table 9.4.

It is evident from Table 9.4 that purchase decision-makers' income had an effect independent from their ethnic group on their satisfaction with life [$F(3)=19.42, p<0.001$]. There was also no interaction effect between their ethnic group and their income ($p=0.480$). Notably, the independent effect of purchase decision-makers' ethnic group is now not significant at the 0.01 level ($p=0.044$). The effect of purchase decision-makers' income on their life satisfaction therefore did not depend on the ethnic group to which they belonged. Purchase decision-makers across all ethnic groups were less satisfied with their lives the lower their incomes were (see Fig. 9.2).

Table 9.4 ANOVA results for the effect of ethnic group and income on satisfaction with life

Source	df	F	Significance
Corrected model	15	27.311	0.000***
Intercept	1	4,648.887	0.000***
Income group	3	19.424	0.000***
Ethnic group	3	2.697	0.044*
Income group* ethnic group	9	0.950	0.480

* $0.05 < p < 0.01$
*** $p < 0.001$

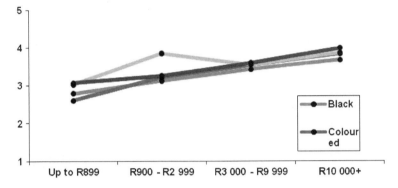

Fig. 9.2 Satisfaction with life of purchase decision-makers in terms of ethnic group and income group

It is evident from Fig. 9.2 that the satisfaction with life scores of purchase decision-makers from all ethnic groups did not differ significantly, especially those from the R900 to R2,999 group and upwards. The only anomaly was that Indian purchase decision-makers who earned between R900 and R2,999 had an unexpectedly high score on life satisfaction, which could be due to random variation. It appears as if purchase decision-makers' income has a noteworthy effect on their satisfaction with life, and this is discussed further in the following section.

The Effect of Income on Satisfaction with Life

An ANOVA was performed to confirm that the various income groups differ from one another in terms of life satisfaction. The purchase decision-makers differed significantly in satisfaction with life, based on their income group [$F(3) = 131$, $p < 0.001$].

To determine amongst which groups these differences existed, Duncan's post hoc test was performed (see Table 9.5).

It is clear from Table 9.5 that all the income groups differed significantly in terms of their satisfaction with life. Purchase decision-makers in the lowest income group

Table 9.5 Post hoc comparisons on life satisfaction between income groups

Income groups	N	1	2	3	4
				Subsets	
Up to R899	542	2.67			
R900–R2,999	783		3.05		
R3,000–R9,999	526			3.43	
R10,000+	306				3.79

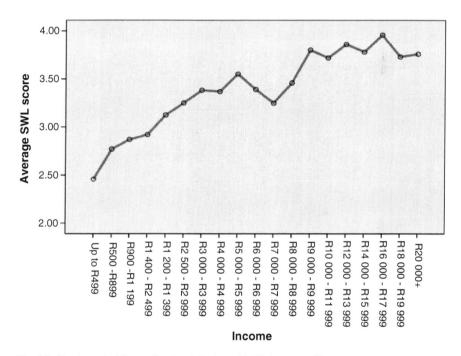

Fig. 9.3 Purchase decision-makers' satisfaction with life in terms of income groups

were most dissatisfied with their lives, and those in the highest income group were most satisfied. Therefore, the lower their income, the less satisfied purchase decision-makers were with their lives.

In the current study, purchase decision-makers' satisfaction with life appeared to rise consistently in terms of their income. To investigate whether there is a point where satisfaction with life flattens out, all groups' average satisfaction with life scores were plotted, as presented in Fig. 9.3.

It indeed appears as if purchase decision-makers' satisfaction with life scores flattened out from around R9,000 – their income consequently appeared not to have a significant impact on their satisfaction with life from this level of income upwards.

Table 9.6 MANOVA: Effect of community size and ethnic group on satisfaction with life

Source	df	F	Significance
Corrected model	20	16.290	0.000***
Intercept	1	3746.952	0.000***
Community size	5	1.147	0.333
Ethnic group	3	24.980	0.000***
Community size* ethnic group	12	2.485	0.003***

* $0.05 < p < 0.01$
*** $p < 0.001$

Table 9.7 Post hoc test for differences in LSM super groups on satisfaction with life

LSM Super group	n	Subsets			
		1	2	3	4
1–3	852	2.76			
4–5	668		3.12		
6–7	423			3.39	
8–10	623				3.73

The Relationship Between Purchase Decision-Makers' Community Size and Their Satisfaction with Life

In light of the fact that the data in the current research was collected from a nationally representative sample, respondents resided in rural areas, villages, small towns, large towns, cities and metropolitan areas. In South Africa, the demographic profiles of people from different communities tend to differ drastically. A MANOVA was consequently performed to determine the combined impact of purchase decision-makers' ethnic group and their community size on their satisfaction with life. See Table 9.6.

The p-value of 0.33 in Table 9.6 indicates that purchase decision-makers' community size did not impact significantly on their satisfaction with life. However, there appears to be an interaction effect between purchase decision-makers' ethnic group and their community size in terms of their satisfaction with life.

Satisfaction with Life of LSM Super Groups

An ANOVA was performed to determine whether purchase decision-makers from the various LSM super groups differed significantly in terms of their satisfaction with life scores. The result [$f(3) = 164$, $p < 0.001$] indicates that the LSM super groups differed significantly in terms of their satisfaction with life.

A post hoc analysis helps to create subsets to assist in identifying where significant differences occur amongst purchase decision-makers from different LSM groups. The post hoc analysis presented in Table 9.7 presents the results from Duncan's multiple comparison procedure used for detecting homogeneous subsets (see Table 9.7).

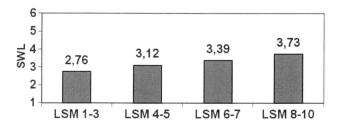

Fig. 9.4 Satisfaction with life of LSM super groups

It is evident from a review of the subsets and the means for groups in each homogeneous subset in Table 9.7 that there were significant differences amongst the four LSM super groups in terms of their satisfaction with life. These differences are presented graphically in Fig. 9.4.

It is evident from Fig. 9.4 that the lower purchase decision-makers' LSM levels were, the less satisfied they were with their lives.

Discussion

Although there may be a myriad of intervening variables, purchase decision-makers who had higher objective living standards reported higher satisfaction with life in this research. Purchase decision-makers from the various LSM super groups differed significantly in terms of their satisfaction with life. The higher purchase decision-makers' level of LSM classification, the higher was their satisfaction with life. Although Diener et al. (2002) point out that it appears that the way people perceive the world is much more important to their happiness than their objective circumstances, it appears from this research that purchase decision-makers' objective circumstances indeed impact on their satisfaction with life. It should, however, always be kept in mind that this relationship is also strongly associated with a person's ethnic group.

Higgs (2003) pointed out that because the LSM is a wealth measure based on standard of living, it can be regarded as a measure of SES. The fact that purchase decision-makers, who had higher objective living standards were more satisfied with their lives, correspond with a finding by Staudinger, Fleeson and Bates (in Triandis 2000) that people's well-being could be predicted from their socio-economic level, both in Germany and the USA.

It also corresponds with Møllers' (2007) observation that a consistent, positive relationship was found between people's life satisfaction and their material standard of living in earlier South African research. Investigating the link between people's wealth and their subjective well-being at the individual level, however, is complicated. This is because peoples' wealth is closely linked to other objective variables that may also influence their subjective well-being. Determining the relative degree of impact of each of these variables can be very complex (Cummins 2000).

Furthermore, the link between people's objective conditions and subjective well-being is mediated by their expectations (Diener et al. 1999). Education may contribute to people's subjective well-being by allowing them to make progress towards their goals or to adapt to changes in the world around them. On the other hand, education may raise people's aspirations and may be detrimental to their subjective well-being if it leads to unrealistic expectations.

Male and female purchase decision-makers did not differ significantly in terms of their satisfaction with life. This relation may, however, be an oversimplification. Additional variables need to be considered in this regard such as gender roles, people's age and which particular component of subjective well-being is addressed. The older purchase decision-makers were, the more satisfied with life they appeared to be.

Frisch (in Sirgy 2002, p. 4) defines life satisfaction as how one feels one's most important needs, goals and wishes are being met in important life domains. The findings on the relationship between income and life satisfaction may be explained in terms of purchase decision-makers' need satisfaction (Maslow, in Sirgy 2002). When a person's basic needs are satisfied, he or she can focus on higher-order needs. The greater their need gratification, the more people tend to move into the higher stages of cognitive moral development. Purchase decision-makers from the higher income group may have been in a better position than those in lower groups to meet their basic needs, which may explain their higher level of satisfaction with life.

Although the LSM segmentation does not include income as an indicator, La Barbera and Gurhan (1997) mentioned that in terms of indirect effects, absolute levels of income or wealth have the potential to affect people's subjective well-being by impacting on how successful they feel, their self-esteem and ability to care for themselves and their family – irrespective of their potential for comparison with others. Higher incomes, for example, make better health care affordable, which, in turn, results in greater subjective well-being for wealthier individuals (Riddick, in La Barbera and Gurhan 1997).

Findings about the relationship between purchase decision-makers' life satisfaction and their community size may require further investigation. A factor which may have contributed to this relationship is whether purchase decision-makers were employed, because people in rural areas are often unemployed. Unemployed people experience higher distress, lower levels of life satisfaction and show higher rates of suicide than employed people (Oswald, in Diener et al. 1999; Platt and Kreitman, in Diener et al. 1999).

Furthermore, some people in rural areas live at a subsistence level (Higgs 2003). Higgs (2007) pointed out that here is a strong correlation (in metropolitan areas) between stress on the one hand and unfulfilled needs and having a boring life on the other. He found that a more varied life correlates strongly with happier, fitter and more fulfilled people. The lowest subjective well-being are linked to poor personal safety, insufficient food, stress and depression, a lack of money for basic needs, a boring life and a number of negative physical health symptoms. These personal problems play a larger role in creating low subjective well-being than people's degree of urbanisation.

In terms of differences amongst ethnic groups, coloured and Indian purchase decision-makers, who were about equally satisfied with their lives, showed the highest level of satisfaction with their lives. Black purchase decision-makers were least satisfied with their lives, followed by coloured purchase decision-makers. White and Indian purchase decision-makers, who did not differ significantly in terms of satisfaction with life, were most satisfied with their lives. Purchase decision-makers across all ethnic groups were less satisfied with their lives, the lower their income were. Purchase decision-makers from different ethnic groups who lived in different communities further differed in terms of their levels of satisfaction with their lives.

Basing her conclusions on the 2002 General Household Survey in South Africa, Møller (2007) points out that 52% of black South Africans were satisfied with life, while 36% were dissatisfied. She found that black people's lifestyles in urban and rural areas appeared to mediate their life satisfaction to some degree, but that people's income and possessions impacted on their life satisfaction in both rural and urban areas.

People from households which had a higher standard of living were generally more satisfied. In rural areas, assets such as cattle, sheep and poultry contributed to people's subjective well-being. Those who were satisfied with their lives came from households that earned more and spent more than others. People who were satisfied with their lives also tended to be better educated.

Those who were dissatisfied came from household in less favourable circumstances and had lower standards of living than others. People who were dissatisfied with their lives were mainly rural and shack dwellers. Their low household income allowed few possessions and assets. Dissatisfaction was also associated with illiteracy and lower levels of education. They admitted that they suffered from loneliness, did not enjoy work and felt that life was overcomplicated.

According to Møller (2007), affirmative action and equity measures such as Black Economic Empowerment have only benefited a small, very affluent, black minority. Furthermore, according to Martins (in Møller 2007), the increase in prosperity that poor South Africans hoped to experience under democracy has particularly not been achieved by poor people in rural areas. Møller (2007) further points out that black people's life satisfaction is partly dependent on different reference standards in rural and urban areas. According to her, blacks may attach particular symbolic significance to material factors which enhance their quality of life. Their income and assets may mean more to them than a comfortable lifestyle – it may improve their self-respect and social prestige, based on their previous life experiences. Their material progress may prove their personal worth in a global society that values consumerism.

Limitations

Because the LSM is based on South African conditions, the results of this study are only applicable to South African conditions. Because it focuses on purchase decision-makers in various LSM groups, the results are only comparable to similar consumers. Due to the dynamic nature of the cultural composition of LSM groups, the representation of various ethnic groups in the LSM super groups, as used in this study, may have changed considerably.

Only the cognitive component of subjective well-being, namely, satisfaction with life, was chosen for investigation in this research. Subjective well-being, however, is a multifactorial and multidimensional construct and no single index can consequently capture it. To fully understand consumer's subjective well-being, researchers should investigate additional components of this construct (Diener 2006; Diener et al. 2004).

Recommendations

In the original SWLS scale, respondents are required to indicate how strongly they agree with the items on a seven-point Likert scale. In this research, a five-point Likert scale was used. The results indicated that this adaptation did not detract from the reliability or construct validity of the instrument and that the five-point version may in future be used with confidence, particularly when less educated respondents are involved. The measurement of people's satisfaction with life in a country with a culturally diverse population such as South Africa warrants investigating the measurement invariance of this version of the SWLS.

Higgs (2007) pointed out the growing trend for consumers to be regarded as people – not just 'consumers' in a market. The term *consumer* distracts from the growing awareness that what is important in people's lives as a whole drives their interactions with markets and brands and other people. Research should consequently present a holistic picture of consumers – marketers need to understand much more about how people live and how they feel about life than they currently do.

Consumption plays an essential role in many peoples' lives (Ganglmair-Wooliscroft and Lawson 2011), and this role may become more entrenched, the more consumers are promised greater well-being in the promotion of goods and services. People who are interested in consumer well-being as such should investigate the relationship between consumers' life satisfaction and concrete experiences in the consumer life domain. In light of the increased interest in transformative consumer research, research in developing countries should particularly focus on vulnerable consumers such as low literate consumers, the poor and their well-being and their experiences in the consumer domain.

Thousands of people globally from desperate poverty who often do not have access to the basic necessities to survive further are exposed to marketing. An understanding of the positive traits – the strengths and virtues – that people such as these possess not to resort to destructive behaviour appears warranted.

Using a deprivation index, an alternative measure of material well-being, which is frequently used in the context of poverty research, should provide a better under-standing of the relationship between people's material conditions and their subjective well-being than indicators like income or wealth (Christoph 2010). Those interested in the well-being of prosperous black consumers in South Africa should focus on the experiences of members of the new black middle class, known as the Black Diamonds (Olivier, in De Bruyn and Freathy 2011). Merely categorising people as belonging to a particular ethnic group may, however, not be relevant in the changing South African environment. Combining people in terms of their ethnic group and language as well as their perceived ethnicity may enhance an understanding of their evaluations of life.

Models of psychological well-being should show an awareness of the existence of various cultural patterns in psychological well-being, and their interventions to enhance psychological well-being must be sensitive to cultural context (Wissing et al. 2006). Neff (2007), for instance, argues that the various ethnic groups in South

Africa have different conceptions of well-being, and that different factors influence their subjective well-being assessments.

To get a complete picture of subjective well-being, researchers should understand the various ways in which people can evaluate their lives. Their personal and cultural values may impact on this process (Camfield and Skevington 2008). A factor that is known to impact on whether individuals and societies believe life satisfaction is an important part of the good life is the cultural value dimension of individualism-collectivism. Investigating the impact of this cultural value on people's judgements of life satisfaction therefore needs to be investigated in future research. But, individualism-collectivism should be investigated as both individual-level and ecological-level constructs. Individual differences on this dimension (in terms of idiocentrism-allocentrism) can be distinguished in larger cultural groups, and relationships between it and subjective well-being on the individual level should increase an understanding of within-cultural variability in terms of life satisfaction.

Lastly, future research should consider the various models of how people create their life satisfaction responses. Schwarz and Strack's (1999) social judgement model of subjective well-being, which focuses on the cognitive and communicative processes underlying people's reports of satisfaction with their lives as a whole, may particularly be relevant in a culturally diverse society.

References

Al-Wugayan, A. A., & Suprenant, C. F. (2006). Examining the relationship between personal, cultural values and desired benefits: A cross-national study. In C. P. Rau (Ed.), *Marketing and multicultural diversity* (pp. 31–52). Hampshire: Ashgate Publishing Limited.

Argyle, M. (1999). Causes and correlates of happiness. In D. Kahneman, E. Diener, & N. Schwarz (Eds.), *Well-being: The foundation of hedonic psychology* (p. 353373). New York: Russell Sage.

Arnould, E., Price, L., & Zinkhan, G. (2004). *Consumers* (International ed.). New York: McGraw-Hill/Irwin.

Burgess, S.M. (2002). *SA Tribes – who we are, how we live and what we want from life in the new South Africa*. Claremont: David Philip.

Camfield, L., & Skevington, S. M. (2008). On subjective well-being and quality of life. *Journal of Health Psychology, 13*(6), 764–775.

Christoph, B. (2010). The relation between life satisfaction and the material situation: A re-evaluation using alternative measures. *Social Indicators Research, 98*(3), 475–499.

Cross, G. S. (2004). *The cute and the cool: Wondrous innocence and modern American children's culture*. New York: Oxford University Press.

Cummins, R. A. (2000). Personal income and subjective well-being: A review. *Journal of Happiness Studies, 1*(2), 133–158.

De Bruyn, P., & Freathy, P. (2011). Retailing in post-apartheid South Africa: The strategic positioning of Boardmans. *International Journal of Retail & Distribution Management, 39*(7), 538–554.

Diener, E. (2000). Subjective well-being: The science of happiness and a proposal for a national index. *American Psychologist, 55*(1), 34–43.

Diener, E. (2006). Guidelines for national indicators of subjective well-being and ill-being. *Journal of Happiness Studies, 7*(4), 397–404.

Diener, E., & Fujita, F. (1995). Methodological pitfalls and solutions in satisfaction research. In M. J. Sirgy & A. C. Samli (Eds.), *New dimensions in marketing/quality-of-life research* (pp. 27–46). Westport: Quorum Books.

Diener, E., & Lucas, R. E. (1999). Personality and subjective well-being. In D. Kahneman, E. Diener, & N. Schwarz (Eds.), *Well-being: The foundations of hedonic psychology* (pp. 213–229). New York: Russell Sage Foundation.

Diener, E., Lucas, R.E., & Oishi, S. (2002). Subjective well-being: The science of happiness and life satisfaction. In C.R. Snyder, & S.J. Lopez (Eds.), *Handbook of Positive Psychology*. (pp. 63–73). New York: Oxford University Press.

Diener, E., & Suh, E. (1997). Measuring quality of life: Economic, social and subjective indicators. *Social Indicators Research, 40*(1–2), 189–216.

Diener, E., & Suh, E. M. (2000). Measuring subjective well-being to compare the quality of life of cultures. In E. Diener & E. Suh (Eds.), *Culture and subjective well-being* (pp. 3–12). Cambridge, MA: The MIT Press.

Diener, E., Emmons, A., Larsen, R. F., & Griffin, S. (1985). The satisfaction with life scale. *Journal of Personality Assessment, 49*(1), 71–75.

Diener, E., Suh, E. M., Lucas, R. E., & Smith, H. L. (1999). Subjective well-being: Three decades of progress. *Psychological Bulletin, 125*(2), 276–302.

Diener, E., Oishi, S., & Lucas, R. E. (2003). Personality, culture and subjective well-being: Emotional and cognitive evaluations of life. *Annual Review of Psychology, 54*, 403–425.

Diener, E., Scollon, C. N., & Lucas, R. E. (2004). The evolving concept of subjective well-being: The multifaceted nature of happiness. In P. T. Costa & I. C. Siegler (Eds.), *Recent advances in psychology and aging* (pp. 187–219). Amsterdam: Elsevier.

Ganglmair-Wooliscroft, A., & Lawson, R. (2011). Subjective well-being of different consumer lifestyle segments. *Journal of Macromarketing, 31*(2), 172–183.

Goosen, D., & Rossouw, J. (2006, November 5). Gefrustreerde begeertes. *Rapport*, p. 23.

Higgs, N. T. (2003). *Are you in (future) shock? The link between well-being and perceptions of the future.* Retrieved from http://www.researchsurveys.co.za/research-papers/pdf/03_futureshock.pdf

Higgs, N. T. (2007). Measuring and understanding the well-being of South Africans: Everyday quality of life in South Africa. *Social Indicators Research, 81*(2), 331–356.

Higgs, N. T. (2008). *The role of race in the South African research landscape.* Retrieved from http://www.researchsurveys.co.za/news-centre/pdf/RoleofRace-2Apr08.pdf

Kasser, T. (2004). The good life or the goods life? Positive psychology and personal well-being in the culture of consumption. In P. A. Linley & S. Joseph (Eds.), *Positive psychology in practice* (pp. 55–67). Hoboken: Wiley.

Kitayama, S., & Markus, H. R. (2000). The pursuit of happiness and the realisation of sympathy: Cultural patterns of self, social relations and well-being. In E. Diener & E. Suh (Eds.), *Culture and subjective well-being* (pp. 113–161). Cambridge, MA: The MIT Press.

La Barbera, P. A., & Gurhan, Z. (1997). The role of materialism, religiosity, and demographics in subjective well-being. *Psychology and Marketing, 14*(1), 71–97.

Lucas, R.E. (2008). Personality and subjective well-being. In M.E. Eid & R.J. Larsen (Eds.), *The science of subjective well-being* (pp. 171–194). New York: The Guilford Press.

Lucas, R. E., & Gohm, C. L. (2000). Age and sex differences in subjective well-being across cultures. In E. Diener & E. Suh (Eds.), *Culture and subjective well-being* (pp. 291–317). Cambridge, MA: The MIT Press.

Mick, D. G., Pettigrew, S., Pechmann, C., & Ozanne, J. L. (2011). Origins, qualities, and envisionments of transformative consumer research. In D. G. Mick, S. Pettigrew, C. Pechmann, & J. L. Ozanne (Eds.), *Transformative consumer research for personal and collective well-being* (pp. 3–24). New York: Taylor & Francis Group.

Møller, V. (2007). Satisfied and dissatisfied South Africans: Results from the General Household Survey – An international comparison. *Social Indicators Research, 81*(2), 389–415.

Neff, D. F. (2007). Subjective well-being, poverty and ethnicity in South Africa: Insights from an exploratory analysis. *Social Indicators Research, 80*(2), 313–341.

O'Leary, B. (2007). Changes in the quality of life of Durban's people. *Social Indicators Research, 81*(2), 357–373.

Oishi, S. (2000). Goals as cornerstones of subjective well-being: Linking individuals and cultures. In E. Diener & E. Suh (Eds.), *Culture and subjective well-being* (pp. 87–112). Cambridge, MA: The MIT Press.

Oropesa, R. S. (1995). Consumer possessions, consumer passions and subjective well-being. *Sociological Forum, 10*(2), 215–244.

Pallant, J., & Pallant, J. F. (2007). *SPSS survival manual: A step-by-step guide to data analysis using SPSS*. Sydney: Allen & Unwin.

Pavot, W. (2008). The assessment of subjective well-being: successes and shortfalls. In M.E. Eid & R.J. Larsen (Eds.), *The science of subjective well-being* (pp. 124–140). New York: The Guilford Press.

Pavot, W., & Diener, E. (1993). Review of the satisfaction with life scale. *Psychological Assessment, 5*(2), 164–172.

Pavot, W., & Diener, E. (2004). The subjective evaluation of well-being in adulthood: Findings and implications. *Ageing International, 29*(2), 113–115.

Pavot, W., & Diener, E. (2008). The satisfaction with life scale and the emerging construct of life satisfaction. *The Journal of Positive Psychology, 3*(2), 137–152.

Richins, M. L. (2004). The material values scale: Measurement properties and development of a short form. *Journal of Consumer Research, 31*(1), 209–219.

Schiffman, L. G., & Kanuk, L. L. (2007). *Consumer behavior* (9th ed.). Upper-Saddle River: Pearson Prentice-Hall.

Schimmack, U. (2008). The structure of subjective well-being. In M. E. Eid & R. J. Larsen (Eds.), *The science of subjective well-being* (pp. 97–123). New York: The Guilford Press.

Schmuck, P., & Sheldon, K. M. (2001). Life goals and well-being: To the frontiers of life goal research. In P. Schmuck & K. M. Sheldon (Eds.), *Life goals and well-being – Towards a positive psychology of human striving* (pp. 1–17). Göttingen: Hofgrefe & Huber Publishers.

Schwarz, N., & Strack, F. (1999). Reports of subjective well-being: Judgmental processes and their methodological implications. In D. Kahneman, E. Diener, & N. Schwarz (Eds.), *Well-being: The foundations of hedonic psychology* (pp. 61–84). New York: Russell Sage Foundation.

Shevel, A., & Klein, M. (2008, February 24). SA's wealth distribution 'is a timebomb'. *Sunday Times Business Times*, p. 8.

Sirgy, M. J. (2002). *The psychology of quality of life*. Dordrecht: Kluwer Academic Publishers.

Sirgy, M. J., & Lee, D. (2008). Well-being marketing: An ethical business philosophy for consumer goods firms. *Journal of Business Ethics, 77*(4), 377–403.

South African Research Foundation (SAARF). http://www.saarf.co.za. Accessed on 30 June 2012.

Tranter, K. A., Stuart-Hill, T., & Parker, J. (2009). *An introduction to revenue management for the hospitality industry – Principles and practices for the real world*. Upper Saddle River: Pearson Education, Inc.

Triandis, H. C. (2000). Cultural syndromes and subjective well-being. In E. Diener & E. Suh (Eds.), *Culture and subjective well-being* (pp. 13–36). Cambridge, MA: The MIT Press.

Tucker, K. L., Ozer, D. J., Lyubomirski, S., & Boehm, J. K. (2006). Testing for measurement invariance in the satisfaction with life scale: A comparison of Russians and North Americans. *Social Indicators Research, 78*(2), 341–360.

Van de Vijver, F., & Leung, K. (1997). *Methods and data analysis for cross-cultural research*. Thousand Oaks: Sage Publications, Inc.

Wierzbicka, A. (2009). What makes a good life? A cross-linguistic and cross-cultural perspective. *The Journal of Positive Psychology, 4*(4), 260–272.

Wissing, M. P., & Van Eeden, C. (2002). Empirical clarification of the nature of psychological well-being. *South African Journal of Psychology, 32*, 32–44.

Wissing, M. P., Wissing, J. A. B., Du Toit, M. M., & Temane, Q. M. (2006). Patterns of psychological well-being and satisfaction with life in cultural context. In A. Delle Fave (Ed.), *Dimensions of well-being: Research and intervention* (pp. 14–33). Milano: Franco Angeli.

Chapter 10
Circumstances of Well-Being Among Czech College Students

Iva Šolcová and Vladimír Kebza

Introduction

In spite of the plurality of views and approaches (usual in psychology) regarding the definition of well-being, scholars basically agree on it being a long-lasting emotional condition which reflects the level of satisfaction of an individual with his/her life. Also, there is a general agreement that well-being needs to be understood and measured by way of its cognitive, emotional, social and cultural components, as well as the fact that well-being is characterized by consistence across different situations and stability over time (for review, see Diener et al. 1999, 2006; Keyes et al. 2002).

The present study concentrates on the issue of well-being as perceived by Czech college students.

Method

The research was undertaken within an international study of cross-cultural comparison of college students' well-being, initiated and coordinated by Cecilia Cheng from the University of Hong Kong.

The study was funded by the Czech Science Foundation, project no. P407/11/2226.

I. Šolcová (✉)
Institute of Psychology, Academy of Sciences of the Czech Republic, Prague, Czech Republic

Politických vězňů 7, Praha 1, 110 00, Czech Republic
e-mail: solcova@praha.psu.cas.cz

V. Kebza
National Institute of Public Health, Prague

Šrobárova 49, Praha 10, 100 00, Czech Republic

H.H. Knoop and A. Delle Fave (eds.), *Well-Being and Cultures: Perspectives from Positive Psychology*, Cross-Cultural Advancements in Positive Psychology 3, DOI 10.1007/978-94-007-4611-4_10, © Springer Science+Business Media Dordrecht 2013

Sample

The study included 535 Czech students aged 19–29 (average age of 20.4; 36.4% males, 63.6% females). The students involved were from the Faculty of Arts and the College of Education at Charles University and the Faculty of Economics and Management at the Czech University of Life Sciences. At the beginning of the research, the respondents confirmed their informed consent by signatures. The research was conducted anonymously, and the respondents only provided their age and gender.

Materials

The questionnaire battery has been compiled by a coordination centre in Hong Kong. The variables were selected to capture four levels of personality as suggested in Sheldon's (2004) multiple levels of personality model, namely, self/narratives, goals/motives, traits/dispositions and universal needs. The authors of the present study translated the questionnaires for which Czech versions were not available. The battery consisted of the following questionnaires:

Satisfaction with Life Scale (*SWLS*; Diener et al. 1785; Czech translation by Lewis et al. 1999). This is a five-item scale; items are evaluated on a seven-point scale. A higher score means a higher level of satisfaction. The Cronbach's alpha amounted to 0.77 in our research. Satisfaction with life was a *dependent variable* in our research.

Schwartz Value Survey (*SVS*; Schwartz and Boehnke 2004). Compared with the Czech 56-item version (Schwartz 1992) authorized by the questionnaire author, the recent version includes one item more, namely, the following: *being unrestrained (doing what I am interested in, what I feel like doing)*. It is assigned to hedonism. The respondent evaluates the items using a nine-point scale, from −1 to 7, where the negative value indicates that the item is in opposition to the values regarded as important by the respondent, 0 indicates the value in question is unimportant and 7 indicates the highest importance of the value assessed. The scales correspond to ten types of values within the Schwartz system, namely, to self-direction, stimulation, hedonism, achievement, power, security, conformity, tradition, benevolence and universalism.

Scales of Psychological Well-Being (*SPWB*; Ryff and Keyes 1995). The questionnaire comprises 43 items to be responded to using a six-point scale. A higher score indicates a higher level of well-being on the individual scales which are as follows: autonomy, environmental mastery, personal growth, positive relations with others, purpose in life and self-acceptance. The Cronbach's alpha coefficients are: autonomy 0.71; environmental mastery 0.67; personal growth 0.57; positive relations with others 0.75; purpose in life 0.68; self-acceptance 0.81.

Positive and Negative Affect Schedule (*PANAS*; Watson, Clark and Tellegem 1988). The questionnaire includes ten positive and ten negative emotions, whose presence in the psychological condition within the preceding month is assessed by respondents on a five-point scale. A high score means a high incidence of positive/ negative emotions. The Cronbach's alpha equalled to 0.79 and 0.78.

Crowne-Marlowe Social Desirability Scale (*CM-SD*; Crowne and Marlowe 1960). The scale includes 13 items, to which the respondent answers yes or no. A lower score indicates a higher tendency to self-stylization in socially positive way. Cronbach's alpha = 0.60.

Self-Construal Scale (*SCS*; Singelis 1994). The scale measures the level of independency/interdependency of an individual's self-concept with regard to the relationships with other people. Independency accentuates the individualistic aspects of self, whereas interdependency, its collective aspects (Markus and Kitayama 1994). The respondent answers using a seven-point scale. A high score indicates high levels of interdependency or independency. The Cronbach's alpha within our research reached 0.62 for independency and 0.60 for interdependency.

NEO FFI (NEO Five-Factor Inventory; Costa and McCrae 1992; for more information on the Czech version and comparison with other translations, see Hřebíčková and Čermák 1996). The questionnaire includes 60 items, always 12 items for each of the five personality dimensions (neuroticism, extraversion, openness to experience, agreeableness, conscientiousness). The respondent answers using a five-point scale. The Cronbach's alpha coefficients reached 0.82 for neuroticism, 0.72 for extraversion, 0.60 for openness to experience, 0.66 for agreeableness and 0.72 for conscientiousness.

Self-determining needs (*SDN: autonomy, competency, relatedness*; Sheldon et al. 2001). Each of the needs is represented by three items whose importance in their lives is expressed by respondents on a seven-point scale. A higher score indicates a higher level of the relevant need. The relatively lower coefficients of reliability possibly relate to only three-item scales (0.44 for autonomy, 0.65 for competency and 0.50 for relatedness).

Statistical Analyses

Following the descriptive statistics, we completed the correlation analysis and then logistic regression. The purpose of the logistic regression was to determine predictors of SWLS score above median.

In addition to the previously mentioned analyses, we also performed explorative factor analysis (EFA) to learn how a latent variable expresses ideas of personal well-being by different authors. The results of the EFA are reported elsewhere (Šolcová and Kebza 2009).

Results

The descriptive statistics of SWLS: $M=21.7$; SD=5.04; median 22 (min=5, max=35).

According to results of logistic regression, the score of SWLS above median was strongly predicted by self-acceptance (estimate 0.20; standard 0.04; Wald 21.5; $p<0.001$) and less strongly by environmental mastery (estimate 0.10; standard 0.04; Wald 5.4; $p<0.01$). No effects of gender or field of study (major) were found. The same holds for the effect of age.

The correlation of SWLS score with those of the individual scales is presented in Table 10.1. The correlation matrix for all the scales is available from the authors.

Table 10.1 Correlations between SWLS and independent variables

Inventory	Variable	r	p
NEO FFI	Neuroticism	−0.43	0.001
	Extraversion	0.30	0.001
	Conscientiousness	0.33	0.001
	Openness to experience	0.10	0.02
	Agreeableness	0.14	0.001
SVS	Achievement	0.04	NS
	Benevolence	0.10	0.02
	Conformity	0.20	0.001
	Hedonism	0.01	NS
	Power	0.05	NS
	Security	0.12	0.005
	Self-direction	0.05	NS
	Stimulation	0.00	NS
	Tradition	0.07	NS
	Universalism	0.02	NS
SCS	Independence	0.16	0.001
	Interdependence	0.01	NS
SDN	Autonomy	0.37	0.001
	Competency	0.38	0.001
	Relatedness	0.26	0.001
PANAS	Positive emotions	0.36	0.001
	Negative emotions	−0.35	0.001
CM-SD	Social desirability	−0.20	0.001
SPWB	Autonomy	0.17	0.001
	Environmental mastery	0.60	0.001
	Personal growth	0.22	0.001
	Positive relations with others	0.37	0.001
	Purpose in life	0.37	0.001
	Self-acceptance	0.68	0.01

SVS Schwartz value survey, *SCS* self-construal scale, *SDN* self-determining needs, *PANAS* positive and negative affect schedule, *CM-SD* Crowne-Marlowe social desirability scale, *SPWB* scales of psychological well-being

Discussion

Links of SWLS with Demographic Variables

As far as descriptive statistics is concerned, the results of our sample (21.7) correspond to average, i.e. 20–24 according to Diener (2006) norms. Comparison of means for the SWLS of Czech students (Pavot and Diener 1993) shows that the mean for Czech students is lower than American college students (with means such as 23.5, 24.5, 25.3) and French-Canadian college students (23.8, and 24.8). However, the mean of Czech students was higher than Korean students (mean 19.7), Russian college students (with means such as 16.3 and 18.9) and Chinese students (mean 16.1).

Potential affectability of well-being by particular fields of study of the participating respondents has not been supported in our research. Similarly to other studies, also the research of our group has shown that the feeling of well-being is not conditioned by gender. The effect of age was not shown likely due to very small differences in age within our sample.

Links of SWLS with Related Constructs

Within the well-being concept by C. Ryff, we have found the highest correlation of SWLS with the scales of environmental mastery and self-acceptance and medium-level correlations with the scales of meaningful life and positive human relations. Logistic regression showed strong association between SWLS and self-acceptance and robust association between SWLS and environmental mastery. As far as causality – both directions are meaningful. The finding contributes to the recent analyses documenting that hedonic well-being (i.e. SWLS in the terminology of Ryan and Deci 2001) and eudaimonic well-being (i.e. SPWB) are related but distinct constructs (see e.g. Keyes et al. 2002). The correlation with both the scales of *PANAS* questionnaires is of moderate level and very similar degree.

Relations of SWLS to the Other Characteristics

Well-being in our research correlates with all the *Big Five factors*, to the highest degree with neuroticism (negatively), extraversion and conscientiousness. According to the assumption by McCrae and Costa (1991), particularly extraversion and neuroticism are important determinants of well-being. Extraversion relates to positive emotions, while neuroticism to negative emotions.

McCrae and Costa (1991) differentiate between the temperamental and instrumental views of the relation between personality traits and well-being. The temperamental view assumes that certain personal characteristics (such as extraversion and neuroticism) are lasting dispositions directly leading to well-being. The other personal characteristics (such as agreeableness and conscientiousness) have, according to McCrae and Costa, an indirect or instrumental influence on well-being, namely, in the way that they lead an individual to encountering specific situations in life, which then influence well-being.

In Blatný's study (2001) of an adolescent group, satisfaction with life (determined by the Bern adolescents' subjective well-being questionnaire) was in both genders related to neuroticism, extraversion and conscientiousness. In a different group of adolescents, Blatný et al. (2004) examined the relation between satisfaction with life (determined by SWLS) and neuroticism, extraversion, conscientiousness and agreeableness.

Hnilica's study (2005a) using SWLS did not confirm the relation of satisfaction with life and extraversion in adult respondents. It did, however, confirm the highly negative relation of well-being and neuroticism. Another study by the same author (Hnilica 2005b) confirmed the relation of satisfaction with life with neuroticism and extraversion in adult respondents.

Sheldon et al. (2011) summed up selected results of aforementioned nationwide study ($N=3,665$ in 21 cultures). The purpose of their article was (Sheldon et al. 2011, p. 10) (a) "...to identify the single best predictor of subjective well-being (SWB) from among the candidates at each conceptual level of analysis" (i.e. at each level of four-level Sheldon's model) and then (b) "...pit the thus-identified best predictors against each other to test the irreducibility of each type of information" (provided by multiple levels). Subjective well-being (SWB) was in their study a composite variable combined from the scores of SWLS and PANAS into a single index. Based on the data of the total sample, neuroticism (that represented the trait level of personality) was statistically significantly (negatively) related to SWLS (SWB).

Well-being is related to *three values* of the Schwartz system in our sample. Therefore, we can add to Ed Diener's hypothesis (contribution of the Ed Diener laboratory... 2005) of happiness being based on values that these are *conformity, safety and benevolence* with regard to Czech college students.

Literature describes that values relating to performance are in contradiction with well-being – Schmid et al. (2005) determined this in German students. Casas et al. (2004) identified a positive relation of well-being and non-materialistic values. Similarly, according to Rask et al. (2002), values like mental balance (composure) and permanent family relationships are among the well-being predictors. Sagiv and Schwartz (2000) did not find in their study of a student sample any relation of well-being (SWLS) and values.

According to the results of explorative factor analysis, well-being in our sample constituted the factor orthogonal to factor based on the values leading to social career, as well as to the factor saturating civic virtues (Šolcová and Kebza 2009).

According to Schwartz (personal communication, 2008), there appear to be no substantial reasons to expect a strong relation between well-being and values. Well-being is influenced, in his view, more by the degree to which the individual manages to work their way to their own value system and protect their important values, rather than the actual value priorities. In his overview of the current status of the value system-based research, Schwartz (2008) described a number of relations between his value system and the varied range of other variables,[1] but he did not mention the relation to well-being. Boski's (2008) research did not find any relation of well-being and the Schwartz value system. According to Hnilica (2007), a core factor which influences the origination and forming of values (and thereby the associated factors) is the process of maturing. An interesting question to explore would be the defining of values associated with well-being in adulthood and older age. We have not encountered any research of this kind in literature.

Sheldon et al. (2011) found, in their summarizing study based on total sample of participants, a statistically significant relation between SWLS (SWB) and self-direction value. Self-direction value represented in the study the goals/motives level of personality. However, self-direction values were not a significant predictor of SWB when the self-determining needs variables were included in the regression.

The independency from the Self-Construal Scale correlates positively with well-being, while interdependency has no statistically significant relation to well-being in the present study. In the study of Kwan et al. (1997), the relation between well-being (determined by SWLS) and independency was mediated by confidence, while in the relation of well-being and interdependency, the mediator was the ability to maintain relationship harmony. Cross et al. (2003) have also encountered the relation of well-being (SWLS) and independency. In their research, however, independency acted as a mediator in the relation of well-being and self-concept consistency.

In the study of Sheldon et al. (2011), independency was statistically significantly related to SWLS (SWB). Independency/interdependency represented "self" level of personality according to Sheldon's model. Interesting effect of culture (indexed in the study as individualism vs. collectivism) was described in the study: *independent self-effect was smaller in individualistic cultures.*

Self-determining needs – autonomy, competency and relatedness – correlate positively with well-being. The relation between well-being and self-determining needs has been recently elaborated in detail by Sheldon et al. (2011). Their results based on the data of total sample showed that self-determining needs (that represented the foundational level of personality) are statistically significantly related to SWLS (SWB). Further analyses showed that cultural individualism acted as a moderator of relationship between autonomy and SWLS (SWB) and competence and SWLS (SWB): the competence effect on SWLS (SWB) was higher in individualistic cultures, whereas autonomy effect on SWLS (SWB) was smaller in individualistic cultures.

The correlation with the scale of *social desirability* (higher tendency towards social desirability relates to greater well-being) is a contribution to the discussion going on for 20 years in writings, of the question whether well-being is a measure of

---

[1] The Schwartz system correlates, apart from other areas, with delinquency, political party preferences, choice of field of study, learning how to use technological innovations, readiness to work, authoritarian attitudes, egalitarian attitudes in relation to gender, creativity, risk-involving behaviour, willingness to help, identification with own nation, etc.

social desirability (McCrae 1986; Mancini and McKeel 1986; Kozma and Sones 1988; Diener et al. 1991). We find the correlation identified in our sample too low for both scales capturing the same construct. Still, we can assume a role of cultural aspect in this question, and the comparison with other countries will be of interest in this respect – especially those where the "tyranny of the positive" is accentuated.

Conclusion

This chapter presents the results obtained from the Czech university student group. The research has confirmed some implicit hypotheses which followed from the construction of the research tool, e.g. the connection of well-being and the Big Five factors, or well-being and social desirability. Also, some relations emerged so far little explored, such as the positive relation of well-being and conformity, safety and benevolence from the Schwartz value system; the positive relation of well-being and the self-concept independence of other people; and the positive relation of well-being and self-determining needs.

References

Blatný, M. (2001). Osobnostní determinanty sebehodnocení a životní spokojenosti: mezipohlavní rozdíly [Personality determinants of self-esteem and life satisfaction: Gender differences]. *Československá psychologie, 45*, 385–392. [In Czech.]

Blatný, M., Jelínek, M., Bližkovská, J., & Klimusová, H. (2004). Personality correlates of self-esteem and life satisfaction. *Studia psychologica, 46*, 97–104.

Boski, P. (2008, July 20–25). *Unraveling the mysteries of the post-communist world: Cynicism that breeds mistrust and unhappiness – A cultural analysis of a cross cultural phenomenon.* In 29th International Congress of Psychology, Berlin, Germany.

Casas, F., González, M., Figuer, C., & Coenders, G. (2004). Life-satisfaction, values and goal achievement: The case of planned versus chance searches on internet. *Social Indicators Research, 66*(1–2), 123–141.

Contribution of the Ed Diener laboratory to the scientific understanding of well-being. (2005). http://www.psych.uiuc.edu/~ediener/Discoveries.htm. Accessed 8 Jan 2011.

Costa, P. T., & McCrae, R. R. (1992). *NEO-PI-R revised NEO personality inventory (NEOPI-R).* Odessa: Psychological Assessment Resources.

Cross, S. E., Gore, J. S., & Morris, M. L. (2003). The relational-independent self-construal, self-concept consistency, and well-being. *Journal of Personality and Social Psychology, 85*, 933–944.

Crowne, D. P., & Marlowe, D. (1960). A new scale of social desirability independent of psychopathology. *Journal of Consulting Psychology, 24*, 349–354.

Diener, E. (2006). *Understanding scores on the satisfaction with life scale.* http://internal.psychology.illinois.edu/~ediener/Documents/Understanding%20SWLS%20Scores.pdf. Accessed 6 Dec 2010.

Diener, E., Emmons, R. A., Larsen, R. J., & Griffin, S. (1985). The satisfaction with life scale. *Journal of Personality Assessment, 49*, 71–75.

Diener, E., Sandvik, E., Pavot, W., & Gallagher, D. (1991). Response artifacts in the measurement of subjective well-being. *Social Indicators Research, 24*, 35–56.

Diener, E., Suh, E. M., Lucas, R. E., & Smith, H. L. (1999). Subjective well-being: Three decades of progress. *Psychological Bulletin, 125*, 276–302.

Diener, E., Lucas, R., & Scollon, C. N. (2006). Beyond the hedonic treadmill: Revising the adaptation theory of well-being. *American Psychologist, 61*, 305–314.

Hnilica, K. (2005a). Vlivy politické orientace, sociálního srovnávání se a osobnosti na spokojenost se životem [Influences of political orientation, social comparison and personality on satisfaction with life]. *Československá psychologie, 49*, 97–116. [In Czech.]

Hnilica, K. (2005b). Vlivy materialistické hodnotové orientace na spokojenost se životem [Influences of materialistic value orientation on life satisfaction]. *Československá psychologie, 49*, 385–398. [In Czech.]

Hnilica, K. (2007). Vývoj a změny hodnot v dospělosti [Development and changes in values in adulthood]. *Československá psychologie, 51*, 437–463. [In Czech.]

Hřebíčková, M., & Čermák, I. (1996). Vnitřní konzistence české verze dotazníku NEO-FFI [Internal consistency of Czech version of NEO-FFI inventory]. *Československá psychologie, 40*, 208–216. [In Czech.]

Keyes, C. L. M., Shmotkin, D., & Ryff, C. D. (2002). Optimizing well-being: The empirical encounter of two traditions. *Journal of Personality and Social Psychology, 82*, 1007–1022.

Kozma, A., & Sones, M. J. (1988). Social desirability in measures of subjective well-being: Age comparisons. *Social Indicators Research, 20*, 1–14.

Kwan, V. S. Y., Bond, M. H., & Singelis, T. M. (1997). Pancultural explanations for life satisfaction: Adding relationship harmony to self esteem. *Journal of Personality and Social Psychology, 73*, 1038–1051.

Lewis, C. A., Shevlin, M. E., Smékal, V., & Dorahy, M. J. (1999). Factor structure and reliability of a Czech translation of the satisfaction with life scale among Czech university students. *Studia Psychologica, 41*, 239–244.

Mancini, J. A., & McKeel, A. J. (1986). Social desirability and psychological well-being reports in late life: A further inquiry. *Educational and Psychological Measurement, 46*, 89–94.

Markus, H. R., & Kitayama, S. (1994). A collective fear of the collective. Implications for selves and theories of selves. *Personality and Social Psychology Bulletin, 20*, 568–579.

McCrae, R. R. (1986). Well-being scales do not measure social desirability. *Journal of Gerontology, 41*, 390–392.

McCrae, R. R., & Costa, P. T. (1991). Adding Liebe und Arbeit: The full five-factor model and well-being. *Personality and Social Psychology Bulletin, 17*, 227–232.

Pavot, W., & Diener, E. (1993). Review of the satisfaction with life scale. *Psychological Assessment, 5*, 164–172.

Rask, K., Åstedt-Kurki, P., & Laippala, P. (2002). Adolescent subjective well-being and realized values. *Journal of Advanced Nursing, 38*(3), 254–263.

Ryan, R. M., & Deci, E. L. (2001). On happiness and human potentials: A review of research on hedonic and eudaimonic well-being. *Annual Review of Psychology, 52*, 141–166.

Ryff, C. D., & Keyes, C. L. M. (1995). The structure of psychological well-being revisited. *Journal of Personality and Social Psychology, 69*, 719–727.

Sagiv, L., & Schwartz, S. H. (2000). Value priorities and subjective well-being: Direct relations and congruity effects. *European Journal of Social Psychology, 30*, 177–198.

Schmid, S., Hofer, M., Dietz, F., Reinders, H., & Fries, S. (2005). Value orientations and action conflicts in students' everyday life: An interview study. *European Journal of Psychology of Education, 20*(3), 243–257.

Schwartz, S. H. (1992). Universals in the content and structure of values. Theory and empirical tests in 20 countries. In M. Zanna (Ed.), *Advances in experimental social psychology* (Vol. 25, pp. 1–65). New York: Academic.

Schwartz, S. H. (2008, July 20–25). *Personal values and socially significant behavior*. Invited address. In 29th International Congress of Psychology, Berlin, Germany.

Schwartz, S. H., & Boehnke, K. (2004). Evaluating the structure of human values with confirmatory factor analysis. *Journal of Research in Personality, 38*, 230–235.

Sheldon, K. M. (2004). *Optimal human being: An integrated multilevel perspective*. Mahwah: Erlbaum.

Sheldon, K. M., Elliot, A. J., Kim, Y., & Kasser, T. (2001). What is satisfying about satisfying needs? Testing 10 candidate psychological needs. *Journal of Personality and Social Psychology, 80*, 325–339.

Sheldon, K. M., Cheng, C., & Hilpert, J. (2011). Understanding well-being and optimal functioning: Applying the multilevel personality in context (MPIC) model. *Psychological Inquiry, 22*, 1–16.

Singelis, T. M. (1994). The measurement of independent and interdependent self-construals. *Personality and Social Psychology Bulletin, 20*, 580–591.

Šolcová, I., & Kebza, V. (2009). Osobní pohoda vysokoškolských studentů: Česká část studie [Well-being in university students: Czech part of the study]. *Československá psychologie, 53*, 129–139. [In Czech.]

Watson, D., Clark, L. A., & Tellegen, A. (1988). Development and validation of brief measures of positive and negative affect: The PANAS Scale. *Journal of Personality and Social Psychology, 54*, 1033–1070.

Chapter 11
Income Is Not Associated with Positive Affect, Life Satisfaction, and Subjective Happiness Among Japanese Workers

Yasumasa Otsuka, Masashi Hori, and Junko Kawahito

Introduction

After the defeat in World War II, Japan faced a serious economic decline. However, the Japanese economy was able to rise from the devastated land so quickly because our predecessors had worked hard to redevelop our country during the postwar years of recovery. Although the gross domestic product (GDP) per capita in Japan in 1958 was only about one-eighth of that in the United States in 1991, there was a fivefold increase in gross national product (GNP) per capita from 1958 to 1987, and Japan became one of the richest countries among the developed countries (Summers and Helston 1991; Easterlin 1995). According to the World Bank's 2010 ranking, Japan now has the third highest GDP in the world, following the United States and China.

Japan has become a rich country; however, our subjective happiness has not changed pronouncedly. Although we have developed many high-quality electric appliances such as televisions, washing machines, refrigerators, air conditioners, and cars during the postwar years of recovery, our level of average subjective happiness in 1958 was almost identical to that in 1987 (Veenhoven 1993; Easterlin 1995; Frank 2005; Kahneman et al. 2006). Moreover, after 1987, even though rapid

Y. Otsuka (✉)
Department of Psychology, Graduate School of Education, Hiroshima University,
1-1-1 Kagamiyama, Higashi-hiroshima, Hiroshima 739-8524, Japan
e-mail: yasumasa-otsuka@hiroshima-u.ac.jp

M. Hori
Center for the Advancement of Higher Education, Tohoku University,
41 Kawauchi, Aoba-ku, Sendai, Miyagi 980-8576, Japan

J. Kawahito
Department of Psychology, Faculty of Human Cultures and Sciences, Fukuyama University,
985 Sanzo, Higashimura-cho, Fukuyama, Hiroshima 729-0292, Japan

Japan Society for the Promotion of Science, Tokyo, Japan

H.H. Knoop and A. Delle Fave (eds.), *Well-Being and Cultures: Perspectives from Positive Psychology*, Cross-Cultural Advancements in Positive Psychology 3,
DOI 10.1007/978-94-007-4611-4_11, © Springer Science+Business Media Dordrecht 2013

changes in the economy have been occurring in Japan, the level of life satisfaction remains almost the same (Veenhoven 2009). Diener and Biswas-Diener (2009) assessed the relationship between income level and life satisfaction by materialism and found that when income level was high, materialism had no effect on life satisfaction, but when income level was low, highly materialistic people were much less satisfied with their lives. To our knowledge, although no data are available on the levels of materialism during the 65 years after the war, we Japanese basically seem to have less materialism because traditionally we have a "wabi-sabi" culture, which is one of our intrinsic virtues, intending to live simply but elegantly. Thus, for most Japanese people, their life satisfaction did not markedly fall and they could maintain good manners and polite behaviors even if a catastrophic disaster occurred and forced them to evacuate over long periods of time. In addition, most Japanese people have a middle-class consciousness based on the Japanese traditional proverb "the nail that is sticking up is ready to be hammered"; Japanese people are not eager to achieve personal accomplishment through beating other people and to express their own happiness compared with Hispanic- and European-Americans (Scollon et al. 2009). For these reasons, the average subjective happiness level might not have changed even if the economic situation dramatically changed.

Several research studies considering the relationship between income and subjective happiness or life satisfaction revealed that, overall, income had almost no relation with these variables. For example, Kahneman et al. (2006) analyzed the data from the General Social Survey and found that whenever annual income was over $50,000, their happiness level was almost identical to that of lower income groups and did not increase much after that. Diener and Oishi (2000) reported the level of correlation between income and life satisfaction in 40 nations and revealed that the average correlation was only .13, which means that income can elucidate only 1.7% of the variance in life satisfaction.

Although the relationships between income and life satisfaction or subjective happiness have been studied in many countries, to our knowledge, these relationships have not been revealed using a sample of Japanese workers. Thus, this study investigated the relationship between income and positive affect, life satisfaction, and subjective happiness among Japanese workers. We hypothesized that income has no association with positive affect, life satisfaction, and subjective happiness even after controlling for potential confounding variables.

Method

Participants

Two hundred fifty-one workers (76 local government workers and 175 manufacturing industry workers) were invited to participate in the study. All participants answered a questionnaire. After excluding 21 participants who left certain questionnaire items incomplete, the responses of the remaining 230 workers (36 women and 194 men) were selected for the present analysis (valid response rate = 92.0%). Informed consent was obtained from all participants before entering the study.

Measures

Annual Income

The level of annual income was measured in the questionnaire with a single item asking, "How much did you bring in annual income last year, including tax?" followed by six choices: "4 million yen or less" (approximately equal to $50,000 or less), "4 to 5 million yen" (approximately equal to $50,000–$62,500), "5 to 6 million yen" (approximately equal to $62,500–$75,000), "6 to 7 million yen" (approximately equal to $75,000–$87,500), "7 to 8 million yen" (approximately equal to $87,500–$100,000), and "8 million yen or more" (approximately more than $100,000).

Positive Affect

Positive affect was assessed using the Japanese version of the Positive and Negative Affect Schedule (PANAS; Sato and Yasuda 2001; Watson et al. 1988). Unlike the original version of the PANAS, the Japanese version consists of eight items in the Positive Affect scale (Yamasaki et al. 2006). Sample items include "excited," "strong," and "enthusiastic." Participants were asked to rate the extent to which they have experienced each feelings right then, at the present moment, rating on a 6-point Likert scale (1 = not at all to 6 = extremely). Cronbach's alpha coefficient was .92.

Life Satisfaction

Life satisfaction was assessed using the Japanese version of the Satisfaction with Life Scale (SWLS), which comprises five items (Oishi 2009; Diener et al. 1985). Sample items include, "In most ways my life is close to my ideal," "I am satisfied with my life," and "If I could live my life over, I would change almost nothing." Participants indicated their agreement on a 7-point Likert scale (1 = strongly disagree to 7 = strongly agree). Cronbach's alpha coefficient was .85.

Subjective Happiness

Subjective happiness was assessed using the Japanese version of the Subjective Happiness Scale (SHS), which comprises four items (Shimai et al. 2004; Lyubomirsky and Lepper 1999). The items include: "In general, I consider myself" with responses ranging from 1 (not a very happy person) to 7 (very happy person); "Compared to most of my peers, I consider myself" with responses ranging from 1 (less happy) to 7 (more happy); "Some people are generally very happy. They enjoy life regardless of what is going on, getting the most out of everything. To what extent does this characterization describe you?" with responses ranging from 1 (not at all) to 7 (a great deal); and "Some people are generally not very happy. Although they are not depressed, they never seem as happy as they might be. To what extent does this characterization describe you?" with responses ranging from 1 (not at all) to 7 (a great deal). The last statement is reverse scored. Cronbach's alpha coefficient was .75.

Covariates

We collected information on gender, occupation (manager, professional, clerk, skilled, others), work schedule (daytime, shift work), employment (permanent full time, nonpermanent full time), smoking status (current, former, and lifetime non-smoker), alcohol consumption per week (frequency), physical exercise (frequency per week or month), experience of positive life event in the past 6 months, age, overtime hours, and sleeping hours.

Statistical Analysis

Differences in demographic and lifestyle variables were assessed using the χ^2 test and one-way ANOVA by annual income level. Positive affect, life satisfaction, and subjective happiness as dependent variables were analyzed by one-way ANOVAs and ANCOVAs controlling for potential covariates to test the effect of annual income groups. All data were analyzed using the PASW version 18.0 (SPSS, Inc., Chicago, IL).

Results

Characteristics of the Participants

Characteristics of the participants and the results of χ^2 tests and one-way ANOVAs by annual income level are shown in Table 11.1. Overall, participants with greater levels of annual income were slightly older and more often men. Among the highest annual income group (more than 8.00 Japanese million yen a year), 78.3% were managers. Shift workers ($n=9$) earned less than 6.00 Japanese million yen a year, and nonpermanent full-time workers ($n=9$) earned less than 5.00 Japanese million

Table 11.1 Characteristics of the study participants and the results of χ^2 test and ANOVA by annual income level

Annual income (Japanese million yen)	<4.00 (n=39)		4.00–4.99 (n=41)		5.00–5.99 (n=53)		6.00–6.99 (n=44)		7.00–7.99 (n=30)		8.00 < (n=23)		Chi-square
	n	%	n	%	n	%	n	%	n	%	n	%	
Gender													25.0***
Women	16	41.0	5	12.2	6	11.3	3	6.8	5	16.7	1	4.3	
Men	23	59.0	36	87.8	47	88.7	41	93.2	25	83.3	22	95.7	
Occupation													150.3***
Manager	0	0.0	1	2.4	1	1.9	3	6.8	9	30.0	18	78.3	
Professional	22	56.4	19	46.3	25	47.2	23	52.3	8	26.7	3	13.0	
Clerk	11	28.2	3	7.3	14	26.4	16	36.4	12	40.0	2	8.7	
Skilled	5	12.8	18	43.9	12	22.6	1	2.3	0	0.0	0	0.0	
Others	1	2.6	0	0.0	1	1.9	1	2.3	1	3.3	0	0.0	
Work schedule													16.6***
Daytime	38	97.4	40	97.6	46	86.8	44	100.0	30	100.0	23	100.0	
Shift work	1	2.6	1	2.4	7	13.2	0	0.0	0	0.0	0	0.0	
Employment													34.9***
Permanent full time	31	79.5	40	97.6	53	100.0	44	100.0	30	100.0	23	100.0	
Nonpermanent full time	8	20.5	1	2.4	0	0.0	0	0.0	0	0.0	0	0.0	
Smoking status													18.6*
Current smoker	27	69.2	20	48.6	22	41.5	30	68.2	14	46.7	10	43.5	
Former smoker	2	5.1	7	17.1	13	24.5	8	18.2	9	30.0	7	30.4	
Lifetime nonsmoker	10	25.6	14	34.1	18	34.0	6	13.6	7	23.3	6	26.1	
Alcohol consumption													17.4
≥6 days/week	4	10.3	10	24.4	17	32.1	18	40.9	9	30.0	10	43.5	
3–5 days/week	5	12.8	8	19.5	8	15.1	5	11.4	5	16.7	1	4.3	
1–2 days/week	8	20.5	9	22.0	10	18.9	9	20.5	6	20.0	4	17.4	
Rarely	22	56.4	14	34.1	18	34.0	12	27.3	10	33.3	8	34.8	

(continued)

Table 11.1 (continued)

Annual income (Japanese million yen)	<4.00 (n=39)		4.00–4.99 (n=41)		5.00–5.99 (n=53)		6.00–6.99 (n=44)		7.00–7.99 (n=30)		8.00 < (n=23)		Chi-square
	n	%	n	%	n	%	n	%	n	%	n	%	
Physical exercise													14.0
Almost everyday	3	7.7	4	9.8	6	11.3	4	9.1	3	10.0	1	4.3	
3–4 days/week	7	17.5	6	14.0	6	11.3	7	15.6	1	3.3	2	8.7	
1–2 days/week	4	10.3	8	19.5	15	28.3	9	20.5	5	16.7	6	26.1	
1–3 days/month	13	33.3	12	29.3	11	20.8	9	20.5	9	30.0	4	17.4	
None	12	30.8	11	26.8	15	28.3	15	34.1	12	40.0	10	43.5	
Experience of positive life event in the past 6 months													3.1
Yes	29	74.4	29	70.7	41	77.4	31	70.5	18	60.0	17	73.9	
No	10	25.6	12	29.3	12	22.6	13	29.5	12	40.0	6	26.1	
	M	SD	M	SD	M	SD	M	SD	M	SD	M	SD	F-value
Age (years)	30.1	9.1	36.6	7.6	42.6	7.5	45.0	6.5	48.9	6.7	49.1	5.8	35.1***
Overtime hours	14.2	25.3	21.0	35.9	12.8	12.1	15.7	15.7	16.6	19.5	24.7	22.9	1.3
Sleeping hours	6.4	1.2	6.3	0.8	6.4	0.8	6.2	0.9	6.4	0.9	6.2	0.9	0.5

*$p < .05$; *** $p < .001$

yen a year. Among the lowest annual income group (less than 4.00 Japanese million yen a year), 69.2% currently smoked. No significant differences were found in alcohol consumption, physical exercise, experience of positive life event in the past 6 months, overtime hours, and sleeping hours among the workers with different levels of annual income.

Relationships Between Level of Annual Income and Positive Affect, Life Satisfaction, and Subjective Happiness

We examined whether the level of annual income was associated with positive affect, life satisfaction, and subjective happiness. The results of ANOVAs showed no significant main effect of annual income level on the scores of positive affect, life satisfaction, and subjective happiness (Table 11.2). Also, after controlling for age, gender, occupation, work schedule, employment, and smoking status, the ANCOVAs showed no significant main effect of annual income level on the scores of positive affect, life satisfaction, and subjective happiness (Table 11.3).

Discussion

Income had no association with positive affect, life satisfaction, and subjective happiness among Japanese workers. These associations were almost identical when controlling for other potential confounding variables such as age, gender, occupation, work schedule, employment, and smoking status. Thus, our results provide additional evidence to validate the lack of associations between income and positive affect, life satisfaction, and subjective happiness.

Diener et al. (2010) analyzed the massive survey of 132 countries with more than 130,000 participants conducted by Gallup Organization from 2005 to 2006 and found that relative income had significant but small positive correlation with positive feelings ($r=.11$). For European countries, no significant relationships between income and satisfaction with work or main activity were found, except for Southern European countries, such as Spain, Greece, Italy, and Portugal (Pedersen and Schmidt 2011). Many previous studies revealed that no significant relationships between income and positive affect, life satisfaction, or subjective happiness could be found, especially among industrialized countries. Since Japan is now one of the most industrialized countries in the world, we could not find any significant associations between income and positive affect, life satisfaction, and subjective happiness.

Several reasons that the relationships between income and positive affect, life satisfaction, and subjective happiness could not be shown in this study should be noted. First, participants with higher annual income were more often managers.

Table 11.2 Positive affect, life satisfaction, and subjective happiness of the participants by annual income level and the results of ANOVA

Annual income (Japanese million yen)	<4.00 (n=39)		4.00–4.99 (n=41)		5.00–5.99 (n=53)		6.00–6.99 (n=44)		7.00–7.99 (n=30)		8.00 < (n=23)		F-value
	M	SD	M	SD	M	SD	M	SD	M	SD	M	SD	
Positive affect	24.9	7.2	23.9	7.6	25.5	6.8	25.8	7.7	24.7	6.4	28.7	7.4	1.4
Life satisfaction	17.2	5.8	18.4	5.0	18.2	5.4	19.8	4.4	19.1	5.4	19.2	4.6	1.3
Subjective happiness	17.9	4.4	17.3	3.6	17.7	3.2	18.7	2.9	18.6	3.2	18.1	3.4	1.0

Note: M mean, SD standard deviation

Table 11.3 Adjusted means and standard errors of the scores for positive affect, life satisfaction, and subjective happiness by annual income level and the results of ANCOVA controlling for age, gender, occupation, work schedule, employment, and smoking status

Annual income (Japanese million yen)	<4.00 (n=39)		4.00–4.99 (n=41)		5.00–5.99 (n=53)		6.00–6.99 (n=44)		7.00–7.99 (n=30)		8.00 < (n=23)		F-value
	M	SE	M	SE	M	SE	M	SE	M	SE	M	SE	
Positive affect	24.3	1.5	23.7	1.2	25.9	1.0	25.9	1.1	25.3	1.4	28.0	1.7	0.9
Life satisfaction	17.3	1.1	18.6	0.9	18.6	0.7	19.7	0.8	18.8	1.0	18.4	1.2	0.6
Subjective happiness	17.8	0.7	17.4	0.6	17.8	0.5	18.7	0.5	18.6	0.7	17.8	0.8	0.8

Note: M mean, SE standard error

Managers basically have high responsibility at work. Managers have responsibility not only for things but also for people (Cooper et al. 2001). Cooper et al. (2001) pointed out that for some workers, responsibility for other people's lives and safety is a major source of psychological strain. In the present study, one-third of the study participants were working in the local government where lifetime employment until retirement is completely guaranteed, and the other two-thirds were working at a manufacturing company where many dangerous tasks existed. Thus, the managers in the present study may have felt a high level of responsibility for their subordinates, experiencing high psychological strain and thus repressing the expression of their positive affect, life satisfaction, and subjective happiness.

The number of working hours, which did not significantly differ by income group in this study, is a possible second reason. An increase in annual income generally requires additional work effort, especially an increase in their working hours. In general, long working hours led to higher levels of negative emotions and fatigue (Otsuka and Tatemaru 2010; Otsuka et al. 2009) and lower levels of quality of life (Maruyama and Morimoto 1996) and job satisfaction (Nakata et al. 2012). Although further studies with longitudinal data are warranted to examine whether the number of working hours has a moderating effect on the relationships between annual income and positive affect, life satisfaction, and subjective happiness, the lack of a significant difference in the number of working hours by annual income group may have moderated the relationship between annual income and these dependent variables.

Third, although the result of the χ^2 test did not achieve a significance level of 0.05, participants in the higher income groups tended not to conduct any physical exercise. Active leisure such as physical exercise is associated with happiness (Kahneman et al. 2006). A previous study revealed that the prevalence of conducting active leisure increased as the family income increased in a representative sample of 8,861 Americans (Kahneman et al. 2006); our result was not in line with this finding. Although we did not ask the study participants how they used their personal time, we assume that participants in higher income groups tend to conduct activities that deteriorate their positive affect, life satisfaction, or subjective happiness. As noted earlier, the participants with higher annual income were more often managers. Most Japanese managers generally enter the discretionary labor system; they receive evaluation from the executives for their accomplishments, not for their actual working hours, easily leading to high job demands and excessive engagement in their job. These situations may cause negative spillover and lead to high work-family conflict (Shimazu et al. 2011) and disrupt social harmony which is associated with happiness, especially in Japanese people (Uchida and Kitayama 2009).

Several limitations of this study should be noted. First, since our study design was cross-sectional, we could not identify causal relations between annual income and positive affect, life satisfaction, and subjective happiness. Second, our data were collected from only two worksites, and thus general conclusions cannot easily be made based on them. Third, we did not examine the relationship between much lower annual income and positive affect, life satisfaction, and subjective happiness. Cone and Gilovich (2010) found a relationship between income and happiness when the income level was low. More low-paying workers such as part-time workers should be included in the future study. Finally, we could not exclude the possibility that unmeasured or unknown confounders may explain the present findings.

Considering these limitations, we conclude that the level of annual income may not be associated with positive affect, life satisfaction, and subjective happiness among Japanese workers.

Acknowledgment This study was supported by Grants-in-Aid for Young Scientists (B) from Japan Society for the Promotion of Science (No. 20730445).

References

Cone, J., & Gilovich, T. (2010). Understanding money's limits: People's beliefs about the income–happiness correlation. *The Journal of Positive Psychology, 5*(4), 294–301.

Cooper, C. L., Dewe, P. J., & O'Driscoll, M. P. (2001). *Organizational stress: A review and critique of theory, research, and applications*. London: Sage Publications.

Diener, E., & Biswas-Diener, R. (2009). Will money increase subjective well-being?: A literature review and guide to need research. In E. Diener (Ed.), *The science of well-being* (pp. 119–154). New York: Springer.

Diener, E., & Oishi, S. (2000). Money and happiness: Income and subjective well-being across nations. In E. Diener & E. M. Suh (Eds.), *Culture and subjective well-being* (pp. 185–218). Cambridge: The MIT Press.

Diener, E., Emmons, R. A., Larsen, R. J., & Griffin, S. (1985). The satisfaction with life scale. *Journal of Personality Assessment, 49*(1), 71–75.

Diener, E., Ng, W., Harter, J., & Arora, R. (2010). Wealth and happiness across the world: Material prosperity predicts life evaluation, whereas psychosocial prosperity predicts positive feeling. *Journal of Personality and Social Psychology, 99*(1), 52–61.

Easterlin, R. A. (1995). Will raising the incomes of all increase the happiness of all? *Journal of Economic Behavior and Organization, 27*, 35–47.

Frank, R. H. (2005). Does money buy happiness? In F. A. Huppert, N. Baylis, & B. Keverne (Eds.), *The science of well-being* (pp. 461–473). New York: Oxford University Press.

Kahneman, D., Krueger, A. B., Schkade, D., Schwartz, N., & Stone, A. A. (2006). Would you be happier if you were richer? A focusing illusion. *Science, 312*, 1908–1910.

Lyubomirsky, S., & Lepper, H. S. (1999). A measure of subjective happiness: Preliminary reliability and construct validation. *Social Indicators Research, 46*(2), 137–155.

Maruyama, S., & Morimoto, K. (1996). Effects of long working hours on life-style, stress and quality of life among intermediate Japanese managers. *Scandinavian Journal of Work, Environment and Health, 22*, 353–359.

Nakata, A., Takahashi, M., & Irie, M. (2012). Association of overtime work with cellular immune markers among healthy daytime white-collar employees. *Scandinavian Journal of Work, Environment and Health, 38*, 56–64.

Oishi, S. (2009). *Shiawase-wo kagaku suru*. Tokyo: Shin-yo-sha (in Japanese).

Otsuka, Y., & Tatemaru, M. (2010). Working hours and psychological health among Japanese restaurant services workers. *International Journal of Psychology and Counseling, 2*(4), 65–71.

Otsuka, Y., Sasaki, T., Iwasaki, K., & Mori, I. (2009). Working hours, coping skills, and psychological health in Japanese daytime workers. *Industrial Health, 47*, 22–32.

Pedersen, P. J., & Schmidt, T. D. (2011). Happiness in Europe: Cross-country differences in the determinants of satisfaction with main activity. *The Journal of Socio-Economics, 40*, 480–489.

Sato, A., & Yasuda, A. (2001). Development of the Japanese version of positive and negative affect schedule (PANAS) scale. *Japanese Journal of Personality, 9*(2), 138–139 (in Japanese).

Scollon, C. N., Diener, E., Oishi, S., & Biswas-Diener, R. (2009). Emotions across cultures and methods. In E. Diener (Ed.), *Culture and well-being* (pp. 203–228). New York: Springer.

Shimai, S., Otake, K., Utsuki, N., Ikemi, A., & Lyubomirsky, S. (2004). Development of a Japanese version of the subjective happiness scale (SHS), and examination of its validity and reliability. *Japanese Journal of Public Health, 51*(10), 845–853 (in Japanese).

Shimazu, A., Demerouti, E., Bakker, A. B., Shimada, K., & Kawakami, N. (2011). Workaholism and well-being among Japanese dual-earner couples: A spillover-crossover perspective. *Social Science & Medicine, 73*(3), 399–409.

Summers, R., & Helston, A. (1991). The Penn World Table (mark 5): An expanded set of international comparisons, 1950–1988. *Quarterly Journal of Economics, 106*(2), 327–368.

Uchida, Y., & Kitayama, S. (2009). Happiness and unhappiness in east and west: Themes and variations. *Emotions, 9*(4), 441–456.

Veenhoven, R. (1993). *Happiness in nations: Subjective appreciation of life in 56 nations 1946–1992*. Rotterdam: Erasmus University Rotterdam.

Veenhoven, R. (2009). *World database of happiness, collection happiness in nations, national report Japan*. Resource document. World Database of Happiness. http://worlddatabaseofhappiness.eur.nl. Accessed 21 July 2011.

Watson, D., Clark, L. A., & Tellegen, A. (1988). Development and validation of brief measures of positive and negative affect: The PANAS scales. *Journal of Personality and Social Psychology, 54*(6), 1063–1070.

Yamasaki, K., Sakai, A., & Uchida, K. (2006). A longitudinal study of the relationship between positive affect and both problem- and emotion-focused coping strategies. *Social Behavior and Personality, 34*(5), 499–509.

Chapter 12
Relationships Between Self-Serving Attributional Bias and Subjective Well-Being Among Danish and Spanish Women

Pilar Sanjuán and Kristine Jensen de Lopez

Introduction

Self-serving attributional bias (SSAB) is shown when people explain the situations that happen in their lives in the way that is most favorable for them. Thus, SSAB is defined as the tendency of individuals to explain positive situations with *internal* (the cause of positive situations comes from themselves), *stable* (the cause of positive situations will continue in the future), and *global* (the cause of positive situations will arise in lots of different areas) causes and negative situations with *external* (the cause of negative situations comes from someone or something else), *unstable* (the cause of negative situations will not repeat itself in the future), and *specific* (the cause of the negative situation only arises in that specific situation) causes (Mezulis et al. 2004). SSAB is considered as a manifestation of the self-enhancement motive, which is defined as the tendency to see oneself in a positive way (Baumeister 1998).

Research has clearly shown that the different ways of self-enhancement, including SSAB, seek to protect self-esteem (Campbell and Sedikies 1999). However, currently, there is a controversy about the universality of this motive. While some authors consider that all the manifestations of self-enhancement would be the expression of a universal human motive (Sedikides et al. 2003, 2005, 2007), other authors argue that the protection of self-esteem would be an important goal only in individualistic cultures, where competent and successful people are valued (Hamamura and Heine 2008;

P. Sanjuán (✉)
Department of Personality Psychology, School of Psychology,
Universidad Nacional de Educación a Distancia (UNED),
C/Juan del Rosal, 10 – Ciudad Universitaria, 28040 Madrid, Spain
e-mail: psanjuan@psi.uned.es

K.J. de Lopez
Aalborg University, Aalborg, Denmark

H.H. Knoop and A. Delle Fave (eds.), *Well-Being and Cultures: Perspectives from Positive Psychology*, Cross-Cultural Advancements in Positive Psychology 3, DOI 10.1007/978-94-007-4611-4_12, © Springer Science+Business Media Dordrecht 2013

Heine 2005; Heine and Hamamura 2007; Heine et al. 1999; Markus and Kitayama 1991). Therefore, the best predictor of well-being is self-esteem in individualistic cultures, while in collectivist cultures, the best predictors of people's well-being are maintaining harmony with their meaningful persons and demonstrating adherence to norms, which are their fundamental motivations (Church 2000; Cross and Markus 1999; Heine 2001; Heine et al. 1999).

In relation to SSAB, studies have found that this is displayed in samples from the United States and other Western or individualistic countries, such as Canada or Australia (Heine 2005; Heine and Hamamura 2007), while this bias is reversed, absent, or strongly attenuated in samples from Asian societies such as Japan or China (Anderson 1999; Heine et al. 1999; Kitayama et al. 1995).

Despite these results, the controversy about the universality of this bias is not resolved, and currently any conclusion is premature since both positions are based on studies in very few countries. In relation to Western or individualistic cultures, most studies have been carried out on samples from North America, fundamentally from the United States, while samples from most European countries have not yet been investigated. Regarding collectivist cultures, studies have focused on samples from Asia, specially Japan and China, but countries from Latin America or Africa have not been studied. However, both from the perspective that defends its universality, and from the perspective that considers that it only occurs in individualistic cultures, it is essential to verify both the presence of different manifestations of self-enhancement motive in the various individualistic nations, as well as their absence in collectivistic ones.

Since SSAB aims to protect self-esteem, and this is the best predictor of well-being in individualistic cultures, researchers have also proposed that SSAB could be associated with well-being. In this vein, some studies have found that SSAB is inversely related to psychological distress (Koenig 1997; Sweeney et al. 1986; Wallbridge 1997), while the absence of SSAB or even a reversed SSAB has been associated with psychopathologies, such as depression (Alloy et al. 1997; Mezulis et al. 2004; Morris 2007), anxiety disorders (Fresco et al. 2006; Mezulis et al. 2004), and schizophrenia (Moore et al. 2006; Sanjuán et al. 2009).

However, it is necessary to note that well-being is not merely the absence of psychological distress or psychopathology (Keyes 2002). That is, people who are not depressed or anxious are not necessarily happy or satisfied. Therefore, it is important to investigate the relationships between SSAB and the positive side of well-being, as well as knowing how much this bias contributes to the development of well-being.

A perspective on the study of well-being, which is currently receiving much attention, is one that considers that people's subjective perception of their lives is more relevant than objective indices of quality of life, and thus, well-being is labeled as subjective well-being (SWB). SWB contains an affective and a cognitive component. The affective component entails predominance of positive over negative affect (or positive affect balance), while the cognitive component refers to evaluation of the satisfaction with one's life as a whole (Diener 2000; Diener et al. 2002).

Much research has been directed to explore the different factors that affect to SWB. Thus, it has been found that attributions and expectancies that reflect a positive view about the self and the world play a role on SWB development (Deneve and Cooper 1998; Diener et al. 1999; Lucas and Diener 2008; Lyubomirsky et al. 2005). Other factors such as pursuing meaningful goals, maintaining close social relationships, and having a personality characterized by low worry, as well as using certain strategies to cope with adversity contribute greatly to development of SWB (Deneve and Cooper 1998; Diener et al. 1999; Lucas and Diener 2008; Lyubomirsky et al. 2005; Sanjuán 2011).

According to the evidence and arguments presented above, the main objectives of the current study were to examine the presence and magnitude of SSAB in two undergraduate women samples from Spain and Denmark and to test a model about what the relations among SSAB, positive affect balance, and life satisfaction are like. Additionally, we wanted to explore possible differences on SSAB and both components of SWB among Spanish and Danish women.

Current features of Denmark and Spain correspond with these individualistic cultures (Triandis 2000, 2001). Moreover, previous studies, which have measured the individualism-collectivism dimension, have revealed that scores obtained by both countries are indicative of their individualism (Diener et al. 1995; Kuppens et al. 2008). Therefore, we expected that both samples would display the SSAB. We also expected to find direct relationships between SSAB and affective and cognitive components of SWB in both samples.

Since in previous studies Denmark has already been ranked as one of the happiest nations (Biswas-Diener et al. 2010; Diener et al. 1995), we also expected that Danish would report more well-being than Spanish.

Moreover, in the one hand, SSAB has consequences primarily in the emotional experience (Koenig 1997; Mezulis et al. 2004; Sweeney et al. 1986; Wallbridge 1997), and, in the other hand, it has been found that people use their emotional experience to form judgments of how satisfied they are with their lives (Schwarz and Clore 1983, 2007). Taking into account both findings, we also expected that positive affect balance would mediate the relationship between SSAB and life satisfaction. Specifically, it was proposed that SSAB would lead to experiencing a positive affect balance, which, in turn, would lead to judgment of life satisfaction.

Method

Participants

Two hundred fifteen undergraduate women students (mean age = 22.31 and SD = 2.88, ranging from 18 to 33) voluntarily participated in this study. Of these, 101 were Danish (mean age = 23.41 and SD = 2.85, ranging from 20 to 33) and 114 were Spanish (mean age = 21.34 and SD = 2.55, ranging from 18 to 25).

Measures

The eight-page anonymous booklet contained a short presentation of the study and the adapted versions of the following questionnaires: *Attributional Style Questionnaire* (ASQ; Peterson et al. 1982), the *Positive and Negative Schedule* (PANAS; Watson et al. 1988), and the *Satisfaction with Life Scale* (SWLS; Pavot and Diener 1993) (Cabañero et al. 2004; Jensen de López 2010; Sandin et al. 1999; Sanjuán and Magallares 2006).

The *ASQ* is a self-report instrument containing 12 hypothetical events, six negative and six positive. For each situation, subjects decide what they believe would be the major cause of the event, and they indicate on three 7-point scales the extent to which they would attribute these events to internal, stable, and global causes. A rating of "1" on the scales indicates an external (totally due to other people or circumstances), unstable (the cause will never again be present), and specific (the cause influences just this particular situation) attribution, while on the other extreme, a "7" reflects an internal (totally due to me), stable (the cause will always be present), and global (the cause influences other situations in my life) attribution.

Two composite scores, for positive and negative events, were calculated, which respectively correspond to attributional style for positive and negative situations. These scores were computed by averaging the items of positive or negative situations, respectively. Alpha coefficients for composite positive and negative were: .74 and .75, respectively, for the total sample; .72 and .70, respectively, for the Danish sample; and .76 and .73, respectively, for the Spanish sample.

A self-serving attributional bias score was calculated by subtracting attributions for negative outcomes from attributions for positive outcomes. This score provides an index of the direction or valence (negative or positive) of bias as well as its magnitude. A positive score reflects an SSAB (or stronger attributions for positive than for negative outcomes), a negative score reflects a self-derogating bias (or weaker attributions for positive than for negative outcomes), and a score of 0 reflects even-handedness.

The *PANAS* is a 20-item measure that evaluates two dimensions: positive affect (10 items) and negative affect (10 items). The response scale was a 5-point Lykert type. Respondents were asked to report how they usually felt. Positive and negative affect scores were computed by averaging items of positive or negative affect scales, respectively. Alpha coefficients for positive and negative affect were: .81 and .82, respectively, for the total sample; .79 and .78, respectively, for the Danish sample; and .84 and .87, respectively, for the Spanish sample.

The negative affect score was subtracted from the positive affect score to obtain a measure of positive affect balance. Thus, a positive score reflects a predominance of positive over negative affect, while a negative score reflects a predominance of negative over positive affect. One advantage of positive affect balance over one-dimensional measures of positive and negative affect is that it controls for extremity biases (Schimmack and Diener 1997).

The *SWLS* is a 5-item measure of global life satisfaction, or a person's satisfaction with life as a whole, rather than any specific domain. Respondents are asked to

Table 12.1 Descriptive statistics on analyzed variables by nationality

		Danish ($n=101$)	Spanish ($n=114$)	Total ($n=215$)
SSAB	*Mean*	0.90	1.19	1.05
	SD	0.76	0.77	0.78
Positive affect balance	*Mean*	1.71	1.41	1.55
	SD	0.76	0.90	0.85
Life satisfaction	*Mean*	6.08	4.78	5.39
	SD	0.93	0.97	1.15

Note: SSAB = self-serving attributional bias; positive affect balance = positive affect − negative affect

rate the extent of their agreement to these items across a 7-point Lykert-type scale ranging from 1 (strongly disagree) to 7 (strongly agree). A score was computed by averaging the 5 items of scale. Higher scores on the SWLS reflect greater life satisfaction. In the current study, alpha coefficients were: .89 for the total sample, .82 for the Danish sample, and .85 for the Spanish sample.

Procedure

The people who agreed to participate in the study were asked to fill out the three described measures (all in the same order) in the classroom before a course. It took about 20 min to complete the questionnaires. When participants had finished, one of the researchers gave them a brief report about the proposals and goals of the study.

Results

The means and standard deviations on analyzed variables by group according to nationality can be seen in Table 12.1. Both groups showed positive scores, demonstrating the presence of SSAB.

In order to compare our results with those obtained in other samples, the SSAB effect size was also computed using d, which is defined as the mean internal, stable, and global attribution for positive situations minus the mean for negative situations, divided by the mean standard deviation (Hedges 1981). The d values were 1.58 and 1.98 for Danish and Spanish samples, respectively. These magnitudes are similar to or greater than those found in samples of healthy individuals from the United States and other Western countries like Canada or Australia (Mezulis et al. 2004).

To explore possible differences on analyzed variables between Danish and Spanish women, analyses of variance for each of the three dependent measures (SSAB, positive affect balance, and life satisfaction) were conducted with nationality (Danish vs. Spanish) as the between-subject factor. Etas partial squared (η_p^2) were

Table 12.2 Correlations between analyzed variables

	1	2	3
1. SSAB	–	.24*	.17[a]
2. Positive affect balance	.34**	–	.59**
3. Life satisfaction	.21*	.45**	–

Notes: *SSAB* = self-serving attributional bias; positive affect balance = positive affect – negative affect
Correlations above the diagonal correspond to the Danish sample, while those below the diagonal correspond to the Spanish sample
*$p < .01$; **$p < .001$
[a]$p = .09$

also calculated as indices of effect size. These analyses revealed that there were significant differences among the Danish and the Spanish on the three analyzed variables. Thus, Spanish women displayed a stronger bias than Danish women ($F = 7.89$, $df = 1,213$, $p < .005$, $\eta_p^2 = .04$), while Danish women reported a more positive affect balance ($F = 6.55$, $df = 1,213$, $p < .01$, $\eta_p^2 = .03$) and greater life satisfaction ($F = 101.55$, $df = 1,213$, $p < .001$, $\eta_p^2 = .32$) than Spanish women.

Since there were differences in analyzed variables, Pearson correlations between SSAB and two components of SWB were calculated separately. As can be seen in Table 12.2, SSAB correlated with both SWB components, although correlation with life satisfaction in the Danish sample reached only marginal significance.

To test whether positive affect balance was a mediating variable linking SSAB to judgment of life satisfaction, procedures outlined by Baron and Kenny (1986) were followed. The requirement to test the mediation is that the predictor (SSAB), the criterion (life satisfaction), and the mediating variables (positive affect balance) are significantly correlated. As we have seen, all correlations were statistically significant except that between SSAB and life satisfaction in the Danish sample, which reached only marginal significance. However, and since this correlation is bordering on significance, we decided to test the mediating effect. Mediation occurs if the inclusion of the mediating variable into the regression equation decreases the relationship between the predictor and criterion variables, and if, moreover, criterion variable is still predicted by mediating variable. The results of the two hierarchical regression analyses for Danish and Spanish samples have been summarized in Tables 12.3 and 12.4, respectively.

According to these results, positive affect balance mediates the relationship between SSAB and life satisfaction in both samples.

To test whether the reduction in the relationship between predictor and criteria variables is significant, when the mediating variable is included in the regression model, the procedure outlined by Sobel (1988) was followed. Since *Z*s obtained through Sobel test were 2.47 and 2.75 (all $p < 0.01$) for Danish and Spanish samples, respectively, it can be said that the relationship between SSAB and satisfaction with life is significantly reduced with the inclusion of affect balance as a mediating variable.

The results obtained in the two samples can be seen represented in Fig. 12.1.

Table 12.3 Hierarchical regression analysis to predict life satisfaction in Danish sample

Predictors	β	t	ΔR^2
Step 1			
SSAB	.17	1.70[a]	
	Model $R^2 = .02$, $F(1,100) = 2.91$[a]		
Step 2			
SSAB	.02	0.29	.32
Positive affect balance	.59	7.04**	
	Model $R^2 = .34$, $F(2,99) = 26.96$**		

Notes: SSAB = self-serving attributional bias; positive affect balance = positive affect − negative affect

**$p < .001$
[a]$p = .09$

Table 12.4 Hierarchical regression analysis to predict life satisfaction in Spanish sample

Predictors	β	t	ΔR^2
Step 1			
SSAB	.21	2.23*	
	Model $R^2 = .03$, $F(1,113) = 4.98$*		
Step 2			
SSAB	.06	0.68	.16
Positive affect balance	.43	4.83**	
	Model $R^2 = .19$, $F(2,112) = 14.66$**		

SSAB = self-serving attributional bias; positive affect balance = positive affect − negative affect
*$p < .05$; **$p < .001$

Discussion

The main objectives of the current study were to examine the presence and magnitude of SSAB and to analyze their relationships with the cognitive and affective components of SWB in Danish and Spanish women.

In relation to SSAB, the results showed that Danish and Spanish samples displayed this self-enhancement bias, that is, both made more internal, stable, and global attributions for positive situations than for negative ones. Although both samples showed this bias with similar magnitude to that found in other Western samples (Mezulis et al. 2004), the bias of the Spanish women was stronger than that of Danish ones.

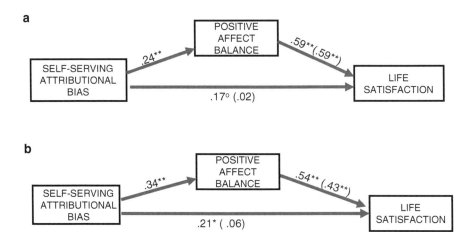

Fig. 12.1 Standardized β coefficients and standardized β coefficients reduced (*in parentheses*) when positive affect balance is introduced as a mediating variable between self-serving attributional bias and life satisfaction [(**a**) model for the Danish sample; (**b**) model for the Spanish sample] $*p < .05$; $**p < .001$; $°p = .09$

These results demonstrate that this attributional bias is also displayed in these countries, and, therefore, they should be considered in theories about self-enhancement. Knowledge about whether people self-enhance and whether this bias reaches a similar magnitude across nations is important for any theory that aspires to understand why individuals are motivated to view themselves positively.

With respect to relationships between SSAB and SWB, our results showed that SSAB correlated with positive affect balance and life satisfaction in both samples. Moreover, we also found, for the first time, that SSAB affects the judgments of life satisfaction through its effect on positive affect balance. That is, the results support that SSAB lead to experiencing a positive affect balance, which, in turn, lead to judgment of life satisfaction. As a whole, these results show that SSAB not only maintains a negative relationship with psychological distress measures, as other studies have already shown (Koenig 1997; Mezulis et al. 2004; Sweeney et al. 1986; Wallbridge 1997), but this bias is also positively associated with direct well-being measures in samples from different nations.

In this way, it could be suggested that SSAB serves not only to protect the individual against emotional distress but also to facilitate well-being development in general. In this way, self-serving appraisals may be a strategy that many people tend to use to maintain psychological homeostasis, especially when faced with difficult stressful situations.

Likewise, previous studies have found that Danish people reported one of the highest levels of well-being (Biswas-Diener et al. 2010; Diener et al. 1995); our results also showed that Danish women subjectively feel that they enjoy greater well-being than Spanish women. Beyond confirming these results, further studies should identify not only what factors facilitate the achievement of these high levels of happiness but also how much each contributes to happiness when all factors are considered together. Knowledge of what factors influence the well-being and how strong these influences are would allow us to develop the accurate well-being promotion programs.

Currently, we know that well-being is achieved by the influence of different factors. Making attributions in a healthy way is an important factor in the development of well-being (Deneve and Cooper 1998; Diener et al. 1999). As noted above, the achievement of meaningful goals, the maintenance of good relationships, the use of adaptive coping strategies, and the low experience of worries are the most important factors that contribute to the development of well-being (Deneve and Cooper 1998; Diener et al. 1999; Lucas and Diener 2008; Lyubomirsky et al. 2005; Sanjuán 2011). Research must be directed to study all these factors together to determine the relative contribution of each of them, and whether this contribution is different depending on the characteristics of nations.

Besides these features, which are more or less under personal control, other factors such as genetic or life circumstances contribute to the development of well-being (Lyubomirsky et al. 2005; Myers 2000). In relation to life circumstances, there is a current trend, supported by some studies (Biswas-Diener 2008; Biswas-Diener et al. 2010; Deaton 2008; Diener and Biswas-Diener 2002; Diener et al. 1995), which considers that some socioeconomic variables such as unemployment rate, access to health and education systems, respect for human right, equality, or income have certain influence in well-being, emphasizing thus that its development not only depends on individuals but also on social institutions. These socioeconomic factors would affect the well-being by providing the means to fulfill basic needs and by allowing individuals to make progress toward their goals, which, as we have previously indicated, have an important contribution to well-being.

In this sense, beyond the different psychological factors that affect the development of SWB, which will be the goal of future studies, Denmark and Spain differ on various objective socioeconomic indices, which could explain, at least in part, the differences obtained here on SWB. Thus, even in 2008, which was when the data are collected, all socioeconomic indices (such as gross domestic product per inhabitant, unemployment rate, budget surplus, deficit of gross domestic product, public health, and education systems budget) were better in Denmark than in Spain (Eurostat 2008).

In support to our hypothesis about the possibility that availability of socioeconomic resources can explain the high levels of Danish people well-being, some research suggests that in Denmark, wealth is more equally distributed than in other rich countries (Biswas-Diener et al. 2010). The availability of socioeconomic resources along with greater access to them could explain why Danish people report more well-being than other wealthier countries, such as the United States (Diener et al. 1995), and that in Denmark there are no differences in well-being between the poorest and the richest people (Biswas-Diener et al. 2010).

This study was subject to some limitations that deserve mention. First, it is necessary for the results to be corroborated in other samples that include men, which also allow us to check possible gender differences. Similarly, it is desirable that the results can be tested with samples of nonstudents. Second, it would also be necessary for future studies to analyze SSAB using not only self-reports, which are likely to be distorted, but also more objective criteria. Third, although we have based our study on the results of previous studies which used a measure of individualism-collectivism (Diener et al. 1995; Kuppens et al. 2008), we have not used any measures of this cultural differentiation variable. Finally, longitudinal studies that provide insight into how SSAB interacts with different stressful experiences are needed. This would be a way to know whether SSAB is a relevant factor in promoting psychological well-being and preventing emotional distress.

Despite these main limitations, this study provides new data about the presence and magnitude of SSAB in countries not yet studied and its contribution to the development of well-being.

References

Alloy, L. B., Just, N., & Panzarella, C. (1997). Attributional style, daily life events, and hopelessness depression: Subtype validation by prospective variability and specificity of symptoms. *Cognitive Therapy and Research, 21,* 321–344.

Anderson, C. (1999). Attributional style, depression, and loneliness: A cross-cultural comparison of American and Chinese students. *Personality and Social Psychology Bulletin, 25,* 482–499.

Baron, R., & Kenny, D. (1986). The moderator-mediator variable distinction in social psychological research: Conceptual, strategic, and statistical considerations. *Journal of Personality and Social Psychology, 51,* 1173–1182.

Baumeister, R. F. (1998). The self. In D. T. Gilbert, S. T. Fiske, & G. Lindzey (Eds.), *The handbook of social psychology* (pp. 680–740). New York: McGraw-Hill.

Biswas-Diener, R. (2008). Material wealth and subjective well-being. In M. E. Eid & R. J. Larsen (Eds.), *The science of subjective well-being* (pp. 307–322). New York: Guilford Press.

Biswas-Diener, R., Vitterso, J., & Diener, E. (2010). The Danish effect: Beginning to explain high well-being in Denmark. *Social Indicator Research, 97,* 229–246.

Cabañero, M. J., Richart, M., Cabrero, J., Orts, M. I., Reig, A., & Tosal, B. (2004). Reliability and validity of Diener's satisfaction with life scale in a simple of pregnant women and new mothers. *Psicothema, 16*(3), 448–455.

Campbell, K., & Sedikies, C. (1999). Self-threat magnifies the self-serving bias: A meta-analytic integration. *Review of General Psychology, 3,* 23–43.

Church, A. T. (2000). Culture and personality: Toward an integrated cultural trait psychology. *Journal of Personality, 68,* 651–703.

Cross, S. E., & Markus, H. R. (1999). The cultural constitution of personality. In L. A. Pervin & O. P. John (Eds.), *Handbook of personality: Theory and research* (pp. 378–396). New York: Guilford Press.

Jensen de López, K. (2010). *Adaptations of attributional style questionnaire, positive and negative schedule, and satisfaction with life scale in Danish people.* Manuscript in preparation. Aalborg University, Aalborg, Denmark.

Deaton, A. (2008). Income, health, and well-being around the world: Evidence from the Gallup World Poll. *Journal of Economic Perspectives, 22,* 53–72.

Deneve, K., & Cooper, H. (1998). The happy personality: A meta-analysis of 137 personality traits and subjective well-being. *Psychological Bulletin, 124,* 197–229.

Diener, E. (2000). Subjective well-being. The science of happiness and proposal for a national index. *American Psychologist, 55,* 34–43.

Diener, E., & Biswas-Diener, R. (2002). Will money increase subjective well-being? *Social Indicators Research, 57*, 119–169.

Diener, E., Diener, M., & Diener, C. (1995). Factors predicting the subjective well-being of nations. *Journal of Personality and Social Psychology, 69*, 851–864.

Diener, E., Suh, E. M., Lucas, R. E., & Smith, H. L. (1999). Subjective well-being: Three decades of progress. *Psychological Bulletin, 125*, 276–302.

Diener, E., Lucas, R., & Oishi, S. (2002). Subjective well-being: The science of happiness and life satisfaction. In C. R. Snyder & S. J. Lopez (Eds.), *Handbook of positive psychology* (pp. 63–73). New York: Oxford University Press.

Euro-stat. (2008). http://epp.eurostat.ec.europa.eu/portal/page/portal/eurostat/home/

Fresco, D. M., Alloy, L. B., & Reilly-Harrington, N. (2006). Association of attributional style for negative and positive events and the occurrence of life events with depression and anxiety. *Journal of Social and Clinical Psychology, 25*, 1140–1159.

Hamamura, T., & Heine, S. (2008). The role of self-criticism in self-improvement and face maintenance among Japanese. In E. Chang (Ed.), *Self-criticism and self-enhancement: Theory, research, and clinical implications* (pp. 105–122). Washington, DC: APA.

Hedges, L. (1981). Distribution theory for Glass's estimator of effect size and related estimators. *Journal of Educational Statistics, 6*, 107–128.

Heine, S. (2001). Self as cultural product: An examination of East Asian and North American selves. *Journal of Personality, 69*, 881–906.

Heine, S. (2005). Where is the evidence for pancultural self-enhancement? A reply to Sedikides, Gaertner, & Toguchi (2003). *Journal of Personality and Social Psychology, 89*, 531–538.

Heine, S., & Hamamura, T. (2007). In search of East Asian self-enhancement. *Personality and Social Psychology Review, 11*, 4–27.

Heine, S., Lehman, D., Markus, H., & Kitayama, S. (1999). Is there a universal need for positive self-regard? *Psychological Review, 106*, 766–794.

Keyes, C. (2002). The mental health continuum: From languishing to flourishing in life. *Journal of Health and Social Behavior, 43*, 207–222.

Kitayama, S., Takagi, H., & Matsumoto, H. (1995). Causal attribution of success and failure: Cultural psychology of the Japanese self. *Japanese Psychological Review, 38*, 247–280.

Koenig, L. (1997). Depression and the cultural context of the self-serving bias. In U. Neisser & D. Jopling (Eds.), *The conceptual self in context: Culture, experience, self-understanding* (pp. 62–74). New York: Cambridge University Press.

Kuppens, P., Realo, A., & Diener, E. (2008). The role of positive and negative emotions in life satisfaction judgment across nations. *Journal of Personality and Social Psychology, 95*, 66–75.

Lucas, R., & Diener, E. (2008). Personality and subjective well-being. In O. John, R. Robins, & L. Pervin (Eds.), *Handbook of personality: Theory and research* (pp. 795–814). New York: Guilford Press.

Lyubomirsky, S., Sheldon, K., & Schkade, D. (2005). Pursuing happiness: The architecture of sustainable change. *Review of General Psychology, 9*, 111–131.

Markus, H., & Kitayama, S. (1991). Culture and self: Implications for cognition, emotion, and motivation. *Psychological Review, 98*, 224–253.

Mezulis, A., Abramson, L. Y., Hyde, J., & Hankin, B. (2004). Is there a universal positivity bias in attributions? A meta-analytic review of individual, developmental, and cultural differences in the self-serving attributional bias. *Psychological Bulletin, 130*, 711747.

Moore, R., Blackwood, N., Corcoran, R., Rowse, G., Kinderman, P., Bentall, R., & Howard, R. (2006). Misunderstanding the intentions of others: An exploratory study of the cognitive etiology of persecutory delusions in very late-onset schizophrenia-like psychosis. *The American Journal of Geriatric Psychiatry, 14*(5), 410–418.

Morris, S. (2007). Attributional biases in subclinical depression: A schema-based account. *Clinical Psychology & Psychotherapy, 14*, 32–47.

Myers, D. G. (2000). The funds, friends, and faith of happy people. *American Psychologist, 55*, 56–67.

Pavot, W., & Diener, E. (1993). Review of the satisfaction with life scale. *Psychological Assessment, 5*, 164–172.

Peterson, C., Semmel, A., Baeyer, C., Abramson, L. Y., Metalsky, G. I., & Seligman, M. E. P. (1982). The attributional style questionnaire. *Cognitive Therapy and Research, 6*, 287–300.

Sandin, B., Chorot, P., Lostao, L., Joiner, T. E., Santed, M. A., & Valiente, R. M. (1999). Positive and negative affect scales (PANAS): Factorial validity and cross-cultural convergence. *Psicothema, 11*, 37–51.

Sanjuán, P. (2011). Affect balance as mediating variable between effective psychological functioning and satisfaction with life. *Journal of Happiness Studies, 12*, 373–384.

Sanjuán, P., & Magallares, A. (2006). The relationship between dispositional optimism and attributional style and their predictive power in a longitudinal study. *Revista de Psicología General y Aplicada, 59*, 71–89.

Sanjuán, P., Fraguas, D., Magallares, A., & Merchán-Naranjo, J. (2009). Depressive symptomatology and attributional style in patients with schizophrenia. *Clinical Schizophrenia & Related Psychoses, 3*, 31–38.

Schimmack, U., & Diener, E. (1997). Affect intensity: Separating intensity and frequency in repeatedly measured affect. *Journal of Personality and Social Psychology, 73*, 1313–1329.

Schwarz, N., & Clore, G. (1983). Moos misattribution, and judgments of well-being: Informative and directive functions of affective states. *Journal of Personality and Social Psychology, 45*, 513–523.

Schwarz, N., & Clore, G. (2007). Feelings and phenomenological experiences. In E. Higgins & A. Kruglanski (Eds.), *Social psychology: Handbook of basic principles* (pp. 385–407). New York: Guilford Press.

Sedikides, C., Gaertner, L., & Toguchi, Y. (2003). Pancultural self-enhancement. *Journal of Personality and Social Psychology, 84*, 60–79.

Sedikides, C., Gaertner, L., & Vevea, J. (2005). Pancultural self-enhancement reloaded: A meta-analytic reply to Heine (2005). *Journal of Personality and Social Psychology, 89*, 539–551.

Sedikides, C., Gaertner, L., & Vevea, J. (2007). Evaluating the evidence for pancultural self-enhancement. *Asian Journal of Social Psychology, 10*, 201–203.

Sobel, M. (1988). Direct and indirect effects in linear structural equation models. In J. Long (Ed.), *Common problem/proper solutions: Avoiding error in quantitative research* (pp. 46–64). Beverly Hills: Sage.

Sweeney, P. D., Anderson, K., & Bailey, S. (1986). Attributional style in depression: A meta-analytic review. *Journal of Personality and Social Psychology, 50*, 974–991.

Triandis, H. C. (2000). Culture and conflict. *International Journal of Psychology, 35*, 145–152.

Triandis, H. C. (2001). Individualism-collectivism and personality. *Journal of Personality, 69*, 907–924.

Wallbridge, H. (1997). Self-enhancing illusion and mental health: A longitudinal panel latent-variable structural equation model. *Dissertation Abstract International, 57*(10-B), 6638.

Watson, D., Clark, L. A., & Tellegen, A. (1988). Development and validation of brief measures of positive and negative affect. The PANAS scales. *Journal of Personality and Social Psychology, 54*, 1063–1070.

Chapter 13
Optimistic Attributional Style and Parental Behaviour in the Educational Framework: A Cross-Cultural Perspective

Loredana Ruxandra Gherasim, Simona Butnaru, Alin Gavreliuc, and Luminita Mihaela Iacob

Introduction

Optimists are people who expect good things to happen to them, and these expectancies have a significant impact on their lives. There are different approaches of the notion of optimism. Some researchers define optimism as a generalised belief that good, as opposed to bad things, will generally occur in one's life across a wide variety of settings (Scheier and Carver 1985). Other researchers assess optimism and pessimism as patterns of attributions about the causes of events and infer that attributional styles are the primary determinants of generalised expectancies (Abramson et al. 1978; Peterson and Seligman 1984). Optimism is important for success in the educational area. Previous studies showed that hope, self-esteem and optimism are key protective factors in the psychological development of adolescents (Peterson and Steen 2002), being predictors of emotional well-being and academic performance (Ciarrochi et al. 2007; Leeson et al. 2008).

For a better understanding of the adolescents' outcomes, it is necessary to consider the developmental environment, because individual characteristic could not explain completely the adolescents' outcomes. The model of ecological systems (Bronfenbrenner 1979; Bronfenbrenner and Morris 1998) could be a proper theoretical framework. This model emphasises four concentric, nested systems:

L.R. Gherasim (✉) • S. Butnaru • L.M. Iacob
Faculty of Psychology and Educational Sciences, Alexandru Ioan Cuza University,
Str. Toma Cuza No.3, 700554, Iași, Romania
e-mail: gloreda@uaic.ro; scraciun@uaic.ro; lgim@uaic.ro

A. Gavreliuc
Faculty of Sociology and Psychology, West University of Timisoara,
Str. Vasile Pârvan No 4, 300223, Timisoara, Romania
e-mail: agavreliuc@socio.uvt.ro

H.H. Knoop and A. Delle Fave (eds.), *Well-Being and Cultures: Perspectives from Positive Psychology*, Cross-Cultural Advancements in Positive Psychology 3, DOI 10.1007/978-94-007-4611-4_13, © Springer Science+Business Media Dordrecht 2013

the microsystem in which children are directly involved (such as the family, the school, the playgrounds); the mesosystem – the linkage between the key settings in which children are situated; the exosystem – with the larger social settings that do not involve the child directly but affect the child's life, such as the parents' workplace; and the macrosystem – comprising cultural values and customs influencing the interactions among the other layers.

In this context, our interest focuses on the influence of the individual and ecological factors (at microsystem and macrosystem level) on adolescents' school performance and depression. The individual factor was represented by the optimistic attributional style, the microsystem factor was represented by parenting behaviour and the macrosystem factor was represented by ethnic/regional specific cultural values and customs. The goal of this study was to examine if regional and ethnic differences may determine variation in the relationship between optimism and parental behaviour, on one hand, and depression and achievement, on the other hand. Most of previous research in cross-cultural psychology has conducted interethnic and interracial comparisons (Mezulis et al. 2004; Bodovski and Youn 2010), and less studies have focused on the interregional aspect (Oettingen and Seligman 1990). A novelty of our research is to capture cross-cultural specificities in the Romanian educational context, simultaneously referring to both ethnic and regional criteria.

Optimistic Attributional Style

The attributional style refers to an individual's habitual way of explaining the causes of positive and negative events in their life, according to the reformulated learned helplessness model (Abramson et al. 1978) and its revision, the hopelessness theory (Abramson et al. 1989). People with a pessimistic (or depressogenic) attributional style have the tendency to explain bad events with internal, stable and global causes and good events with external, unstable and specific causes. These people would be more likely to develop depression when faced with stressful situations than people with an optimistic attributional style – who habitually offer external, unstable and specific causes to explain negative events but internal, stable and global causes to explain negative events. Prospective and retrospective tests of the hopelessness theory in adults and adolescents have supported the hypothesis that a pessimistic attributional style increases the risk of depression (Abela et al. 2007; Morris et al. 2008) and decreases school performance (Martin-Krumm et al. 2005).

Recently, in attributional style research the focus has shifted from helplessness and pessimism towards the hopefulness and positive adjustment (Mezulis et al. 2004; Vines and Nixon 2009). Research has provided evidence to suggest that the optimistic attributional style is a significant protecting factor for resiliency (Haeffel and Vargas 2011; Voelz et al. 2003).

Optimistic Attributional Style and the Adolescents' Outcomes

Analogous to the hopelessness theory of depression, Needles and Abramson (1990) proposed the hopefulness model of depression, hypothesising that depressed persons who tend to attribute positive life events to global and stable causes (optimistic or enhancing attributional style) are likely to become hopeful when positive events occur. Empirical research has shown that adults with an optimistic attributional style (alone or in combination with positive life events) were more likely to experience decreases in depressive symptoms than those without an optimistic attributional style (Fresco et al. 2006; Johnson et al. 1998; Needles and Abramson 1990). More recently, the tendency to explain good events with internal, stable and global causes was shown to be an important predictor of psychological well-being, positive self-esteem and effective coping strategies (Cheng and Furnham 2003; Sanjuan and Magallares 2009).

Few studies have tested this model using samples of children and adolescents, and the results were consistent with previous adult studies. Studies reported that both children and adolescences with external, instable and specific attribution for positive events showed greater increases in depressive symptoms across time than those with a more internal, stable and global attribution for these events (Conley et al. 2001; Curry and Craighead 1990; Vines and Nixon 2009). Other studies provided findings that the optimistic attributional style for positive events interacts with the pessimistic attributional style for negative events to predict changes in hopelessness among adolescents experiencing depressive symptomatology (Haeffel and Vargas 2011; Voelz et al. 2003). These findings suggest that the optimistic attributional style may be a protective factor that could reduce adolescents' vulnerability to depressive symptoms, regardless of the number of negative life events they experience.

The association between the attributional style for positive events and achievement has been relatively little researched so far. In the academic domain, it was found that a higher level of achievement is associated with an optimistic explanatory style for positive events (Yates and Yates 1995; Glasgow et al. 1997). However, a high level of optimism may lead to unrealistic success expectations and thus may undermine performance; the phenomenon is known as unrealistic optimism (Armor and Taylor 2002). More research is needed to replicate this finding in different age groups and educational contexts.

Cross-Cultural Perspectives on the Optimistic Attributional Style

Cross-cultural research already revealed cultural differences in the impact of attributional style on depression. Results demonstrated that non-Western cultures' (including China, Japan and Taiwan samples) depressive symptoms were more strongly predicted by the interaction between positive events and an optimistic attributional style than by the interaction between negative events and a pessimistic attributional style reported in Western cultures, including USA, Canada and the Western part of Europe (Lieber et al. 2000). The meaning and the implications of attribution are determined by distinct sociocultural factors. In Western cultures, theories about causality emphasise the individual as the source of outcomes. Consequently, Western individuals prefer to explain their behaviours rather through dispositional than through situational causes. In non-Western cultures, causality theories emphasise the situational factors – individuals often believe that behaviour is strongly influenced by context and social relationships (Mahtani et al. 2004). As much of what is known about optimism comes from studies of North Americans (mostly of European descent), it remained unclear whether the results of the studies also apply to other cultures and populations (Mezulis et al. 2004).

Studies exploring differences across ethnic groups (Caucasian, Latino and African Americans) in the attributional style and the depression level have reported inconclusive results. Some studies found that Caucasians showed a higher level of pessimism and depression (Thompson et al. 1998), and other studies found that African Americans had higher levels on these variables (Stein et al. 2010). Also, studies that analysed the ethnic differences in the relations between the pessimistic attributional style and depression reported contradictory results. While some studies suggested that the relationship may be stronger for Caucasian youth compared to African American youth (Herman et al. 2007), others demonstrated that the relationship between attributional style and depression is stronger for Latino adolescents than for Caucasian and African American adolescents (Stein et al. 2010).

Cultural differences in attributional style and depression were found within the same ethnic group living under a different political regime. Zullow et al. (1988) compared the attributional style of Germans from East and from West Berlin. Results indicated significant differences. Individuals from West Berlin were more optimistic compared with those from East Berlin. In another study, Oettingen and Seligman (1990) found that Germans from West Berlin are more optimistic and have fewer instances of depressive behaviour compared to Germans from East Berlin. Authors claim that the differences in the political administration between West (capitalism) and East (communism) after 1945 could explain the differences in the attributional style and depression.

Although optimistic attributional style is an important protective factor in depression, few studies validated the theory on children and adolescents samples. Fewer studies focused on the relationship between optimistic attributional style and school achievement, although these studies indicated that optimistic attributional style promoted school performance. Considering this evidence, in our study we tested Needles and Abramson's (1990) hopefulness model of depression in adolescent samples. Most of cross-cultural research highlighted racial differences in the relationship between attributional style and depression, but fewer studies analysed the ethnic and regional differences. In this study, we analysed whether the relationship between optimistic attributional style and both depression and achievement was moderated by the ethnic or/and the regional group.

Parental Behaviour

A large body of literature described the impact of parents' behaviour (by the family's socioeconomic status and the social background) on the adolescents' cognitive and affective outcomes (An 2010; Rothon et al. 2011). Researchers studied parental behaviour and classified it in many clusters, such as acceptance versus rejection, psychological control versus psychological autonomy, firm control versus lax control (Schludermann and Schludermann 1970), supporting versus controlling behaviour (Openshaw et al. 1984) and warm/supportive versus hostile behaviour (Repinski and Shonk 2002).

However, from the multiple theoretical models, two dimensions of parental behaviour were distinguished as commonplace – responsiveness/acceptance and demandingness/control. Parental responsiveness (or acceptance) means the extent to which parents intentionally foster individuality, self-regulation and self-assertion by being attuned, supportive and acquiescent to children's needs and demands (Baumrind 1991). Rejection, the opposite of acceptance, was taken into consideration in the definition of parental maltreatment as lack of affection and warmth, high level of negativity, physical abuse, overcontrol and intrusiveness (An 2010; Haskett et al. 2006). Parental demandingness (also referred to as behavioural control) signifies the claims parents make on children to become integrated into the family whole, by their maturity demands, supervision and willingness to confront the child who disobeys (Baumrind 1991). The adolescents' assertion of their autonomy in the learning processes was markedly stronger as they became older (Bernardo 2010). Psychological control is an insidious type of control (Barber 1996; Schludermann and Schludermann 1970) that potentially inhibits or intrudes upon psychological development through love withdrawal, fear and guilt induction, negative affects (e.g. disappointment, shame) and excessive personal control (e.g. possessiveness, protectiveness).

Parental Behaviour and the Adolescents' Depression

Parental acceptance and warmth are related to fewer behaviour problems and a lower level of anxiety, increased self-esteem and active coping among adolescents (Hipwell et al. 2008). On the contrary, parental behaviour such as rejection and neglect were highly related to depression and negative self-referential cognitions concerning one's social worth and esteem (An 2010; Slavich et al. 2010).

There is consistent empirical support for the association between low parental care and depressive symptoms in children and adolescents. Findings for parental control/overprotection were mixed: some studies reported a significant relationship between high parental control and adolescents' depressive symptoms (Garber et al. 1997), while others failed to find an association (Greaven et al. 2000). Researchers demonstrated that parental psychological control was positively related to internalising symptoms, whereas behavioural control was negatively related to externalising symptoms (Barber 1996). Also, the link between psychological control (through guilt, shaming, contingent love and anxiety) and depression was demonstrated (Restifo and Bögels 2009). If parents use psychologically controlling techniques, this increases the vulnerability to internalising problems because this parenting dimension would interfere with the establishment of a secure, stable and positive sense of self and would thus put adolescents at a risk of low self-esteem and depressive symptoms (Michiels et al. 2008; Soenens and Vansteenkiste 2010). Although some research suggests that the socio-emotional support from parents is linked to adolescents' happiness, it is unclear whether such support is likely to exert a strong influence for all cultural groups (Bradley and Corwyn 2004).

Parental Behaviour and the Adolescents' School Outcomes

The differences in the family structure and the socioeconomic status impact on parents' ability to invest in their children's education in meaningful ways. Influential investments might occur early and be largely directed towards ensuring students' success during the elementary, middle and high school years (Charles et al. 2007). Literature suggests that the household socioeconomic status (SES) – usually measured as parental income and/or education – is critically important for achievement (Meneghan 1996; Parcel and Meneghan 1994). Likewise, parents with a higher SES can more easily transmit cultural capital to their children, conducive to educational success (Bourdieu 1997). Living in poverty had direct, negative effects on the cognitive ability and achievement (Pallock and Lamborn 2006). Some studies proved that the presence versus absence of persistent parental support may be particularly important in understanding the academic resilience versus underachievement of Latino students who have a low socioeconomic standing (Bodovski and Youn 2010).

Cultural differences in the effects of parental control on school performances were demonstrated. Within collectivistic cultural systems, where students' academic strivings are construed as being strongly associated with the expectations of one's parents, parental control over some academic attitudes may be considered normative, and, thus, legitimate (Bernardo 2010). The perceived legitimacy of parental control over the learning processes is a negative predictor of GPA in Filipino adolescents. In individualistic cultures, where each individual acts to achieve his personal goals, this positive relation between control and school outcomes is not characteristic. The control may be considered as intrusiveness (Bernardo 2010).

Cross-Cultural Perspectives on Parental Behaviour

Because of the differences in values and in the meaning of parental behaviour across cultures (e.g. parental acceptance/rejection, parental control, corporal punishment), some developmentally oriented investigators have advocated a culturally anchored approach in which research describes the normal range of relationships within a given culture and how those relationships are linked to child outcomes (Bradley and Corwyn 2004; Hughes and Seidman 2002). Therefore, whereas Western – European and American (individualistic) – cultures emphasise academic or cognitive modes of social integration, independence, creativity, assertiveness and autonomy, African, Asian and Latin American (collectivistic) cultures place primary emphasis on social, affective socialisation, interdependence, respectfulness and obedience (Harwood 1992; Nsamenang and Lamb 1994; Triandis 2001; Yang and Shin 2008).

Each cultural orientation (to independence and to interdependence) is built on a set of parenting practices. Thus, child-rearing practices for young children, such as structured meals and separate sleeping arrangements, and day-care attendance in infancy and preschool might be thought of as routines that encourage the child to manage separation, a major step towards self-reliance and independence (Richman et al. 1988). Frequent physical and verbal expressions of affection, co-sleeping, permissive and indulgent parental attitudes and, on the other hand, the tendency to be directive and to exhibit physical control with their infants and to request display of respect and obedience to family and community members are parental practices that encourage child interdependence (Bradley and Corwyn 2004).

The control is a critical and much studied dimension of parenting (Baumrind 1991), but it has a very different meaning from a culture to another (e.g. the Chinese vs. the European American culture). Juang et al. (2007) reported that while in Chinese families parental control is seen as a very positive and caring aspect of parenting, and obedience and deference to parents, spending time with the family and the harmony within the family are highly encouraged, for mainstream European American families, parental control is seen as a negative, or even hostile, aspect of parenting. Bodovski and Youn (2010) found differences between Black, White, Hispanic and Asian parents in some parenting practices. Thus, Black parents were more likely to report the use of physical discipline but also more likely to report higher levels of parental warmth. Hispanic parents did not differ from White parents in physical discipline but were more likely to report higher levels of parental warmth. Asian parents were less likely to report the use of physical discipline, but they also reported a lower level of parental warmth as compared to White parents.

Although previous cross-cultural studies showed ethnical and racial differences in parental behaviour, there are no studies analysing the ethnic differences in the relationship between parental behaviour and adolescents' outcomes. Consequently, in this study we analysed this topic in the Romanian context.

The Present Study

The large majority of cross-cultural psychological studies on parenting, optimism and cognitive and affective adolescents' outcomes are based on ethnic or racial criteria (Bodovski and Youn 2010; Juang et al. 2007; Stein et al. 2010; Yang and Shin 2008). Comparisons were made between populations with different ethnic or racial backgrounds living in the same communities, or in distinct ones. In the present study, we explore the ethnic differences in these variables in the Romanian national context. This aim is justified by the fact that Romania, as a national state, has a long history of interethnic coexistence of the majority (89.5%) with the 18 inhabiting minorities. Their geographical distribution allows the distinction between the mainly culturally homogenous areas and the mixed areas.

Only few cross-cultural studies reported cultural differences on attributional style and depression in populations of the same ethnicity living in different geographical regions (Oettingen and Seligman 1990; Zullow et al. 1988). There are no studies on this topic in Romanian settings. However, Romanian research highlights differences in the attitudes towards the regionally and ethnically otherness. Romanians from Banat prefer the interaction with their fellow citizens of other ethnicities, with whom they have shared the historical experience directly and they felt "closer" with them, than with the Romanians from Moldova "alike with them", brought in Banat by the great wave of mobility induced by the communist regime (Gavreliuc 2011). The differences were explained through various international contexts in which the Romanian traditional regions have developed. The Eastern region, Moldova, is symbolically related to the past traditions, and its history is culturally influenced by the Turkish power domination until the end of the nineteenth century. On the other side, Banat region is associated with the Western modernisation; it takes its social development patterns from Habsburg and the Austro-Hungarian monarchy, under whose domination the region was until the Union of 1918. According to this shared social definition, if the West is the "saving" reference, the East is associated with the prevalence of disengagement manners (Antohi 1997).

Our cross-cultural research covers two geographical regions of Romania – Banat (Western region) and Moldova (Eastern region). We selected these two regions because the Romanian cross-cultural research revealed that they are on opposite poles regarding sociability and orientation of values (Sandu 2003; Voicu and Voicu 2007). Moldova, a relatively homogeneous ethnic region, has the highest aggregate scores in the index of intolerance, which indicates a lack of social capital, restrained relationships, lack of openness at the level of interpersonal and group interaction, institutional conformism and preference for tradition and subsistence values. Banat, a multiethnic region, has the lowest levels of intolerance throughout Romania, which indicates openness at the level of interpersonal and group interaction, preference for rational-secular and self-accomplishment values.

Given that the variables of our study have a socioeconomic determination, we consider it appropriate to point out other such interregional differences (Bourdieu 1997; Pallock and Lamborn 2006). Thus, the comparison between Banat and Moldova (Voinea et al. 2007) revealed many differences in favour of Banat region in three categories of indicators: *economic* (e.g. GDP and labour productivity), *social* (e.g. employment) and *technology* (e.g. research and development expenses and persons employed in high-tech sectors).

In this study, considering as conceptual framework the classical model of ecological systems (Bronfenbrenner and Morris 1998), we explore how the macrosystem variables (the regional and ethnic factor) explain the differences in microsystem variables (parenting behaviour), individual variables (optimistic attributional style) and outcomes (school performance and depression). The first goal of our study was to examine the differences generated by the ethnic/regional factor on the level of optimistic attributional style, parental behaviour and the adolescents' achievement and depression. The second goal was to explore whether the relationships between optimistic attributional style and parental behaviour, on the one side, and adolescents' achievement and depression, on the other side, were moderated by the ethnic/regional criteria.

Method

Participants

Three hundred and ninety eighth-grade students aged between 13 and 15 were recruited for this study. No information regarding their families' socioeconomic status or education was collected. Before adolescents' participation in the study, parents signed informed consent statements. Also, permissions for the study were obtained from the school authorities and from the principals. The participants were enrolled in five public secondary schools. Students who provided incomplete data were excluded from the analyses, yielding a sample of 360. Other 11 children were excluded because they came from single-parent families. The final sample consisted of 349 eighth-graders (173 girls, 170 boys and 6 did not provide their gender; $M = 13.65$, SD = .82) with 94 Hungarian adolescents (all from Banat region) and 255 Romanians (128 from Banat and 127 from Moldova). The participants from Banat region were recruited from three urban secondary schools in Timisoara. The sample included 128 Romanian (60 boys, 62 girls and 6 unknown gender) and 94 Hungarian (55 boys and 39 girls) adolescents. The participants from Moldova were recruited from two secondary schools in Iasi. The sample included 127 Romanian adolescents (55 boys and 72 girls). There was no significant difference in age, $F(2,346) = .44$, ns, or gender distribution, χ^2s < 2.26, ns.

Measures

The Children's Attributional Style Questionnaire – Revised (CASQ-R; Thompson et al. 1998) is a commonly used 24-item, forced-choice questionnaire, developed to assess children's causal explanations for positive and negative events. Participants were instructed to imagine that they have encountered various hypothetical situations. Half of the items in the questionnaire addressed positive outcomes, and half addressed negative outcomes. In this study, we considered the attributional style only for positive events. The higher the positive score, the more optimistic the attributional style was. In this sample, Cronbach's alpha coefficients for positive events were moderate (.36 for Romanian, .43 for Hungarian adolescents from Banat and .31 for Romanian adolescents from Moldova) and similar with the internal consistencies reported in other studies (Morris et al. 2008; Thompson et al. 1998).

The participants completed the *Children's Report of Parenting Behaviour Inventory*, a 52-item version of the CRPBI (Schaefer 1965; Schludermann and Schludermann 1970) designed to assess adolescents' perceptions of their parents' behaviour. We used eight scales for measuring the psychological control/autonomy and acceptance/rejection factors. We selected these scales because the factorial analysis from previous studies reported higher loadings of them in factors (values higher than .80) on the Romanian sample (Butnaru et al. 2010). The scales for the acceptance/rejection factor were acceptance, child centredness, positive involvement and acceptance of individuation. The scales for psychological control were control, control through guilt, hostile control and instilling persistent anxiety. On a 3-point scale ranging from 1 (like) to 3 (dislike), the participants answered each question separately for mothers and fathers. Composite scores were computed for each participant on each of the scale describing both the mother's and the father's behaviour. Factor analyses were performed to compare the construct validity of the scales measuring parental behaviour. Principal component analysis using the varimax rotation yielded, for each sample, two factors accounting from 78% to 81% of the total variance. All eight scales had high loadings, with absolute values ranging from .80 to .91 among Romanian adolescents from Banat, from .84 to .94 for Hungarian adolescents from Banat and from .83 to .95 for Romanian adolescents from Moldova. Considering the similarity in the component structure, the factor analyses supported the assumption that the CRPBI scales measured the same constructs among all groups. For the subsequent analysis of this study, composite mean scores were calculated for each factor describing the parents, taken together. A higher score for these factors indicated a higher level of rejection and of autonomy, respectively.

Depressive symptoms were assessed using the *Children's Depression Inventory* (CDI; Kovacs 1985). The CDI is a 27-item questionnaire that measures cognitive, affective and behavioural symptoms of depression in children and teenagers. Each item consists of three statements graded in the order of increasing severity from 0 to 2. Participants select one sentence from each group that best describes them over the past 2 weeks. Total scores range from 0 to 54, with higher scores indicating greater symptom severity. The CDI has a good internal consistency and convergent validity with other self-report measures (Abela et al. 2007; Morris et al. 2008). The alpha coefficients for the CDI ranged from .53 to .61 across all samples.

School achievement. We collected the participants' grades for each of the eight subjects (Mathematics, Physics, Chemistry, Biology, Romanian, History, Geography and English). The grading scale of Romanian secondary schools ranges from 1 (poor) to 10 (outstanding). The overall average grade across the eight subjects was computed.

Procedure

Questionnaires assessing attributional style (CASQ-R) and perceptions of parenting behaviours (CRPBI) were distributed to all students at the beginning of the first semester of the eighth grade. Three months later, at the beginning of the second semester, adolescents filled in the depression questionnaire (CDI) and reported their average grades in eight subject areas.

Results

Initially, we described the ethnic/regional differences in the adolescents' answers. After that, we analysed whether the relationships between variables are moderated by region and/or ethnicity.

Cross-Cultural Differences

Given that findings from some studies have pointed out the importance of the way the participants' gender interacts with cultural variables on outcome (Watkins et al. 2000), we explored the impact of gender, ethnicity/regional group and gender×ethnic/regional group on adolescents' outcomes. We conducted univariate analyses between gender×ethnic/regional groups on all studied variables. The results are presented for each type of criteria – ethnic, regional and combined.

Interethnic. A 2 (ethnicity: Romanian vs. Hungarian adolescents from Banat)×2 (gender: boys vs. girls) analysis of variance, with optimistic attributional style, perception of parental behaviour, grades and depressive symptoms, revealed a main effect of gender on grades, $F(1,215) = 14.77$, $p < .001$, $\eta^2 = .06$, and gender×ethnicity interaction on the perception on parental control, $F(1,215) = 6.52$, $p = .011$, $\eta^2 = .03$. The analyses indicated that girls ($M = 8.22$; $SD = 1.49$) had higher grades than boys ($M = 7.43$; $SD = 1.41$). Romanian boys reported a lower level of control ($M = 4.03$; $SD = .66$) compared to Romanian girls ($M = 3.95$; $SD = .71$), while Hungarian boys ($M = 3.78$; $SD = .67$) reported a higher level of parental control, compared to Hungarian girls ($M = 4.17$; $SD = .60$). Also, Romanian boys reported a lower level of parental control than Hungarian boys, while for the Hungarian girls there is a reverse situation – they reported a lower level of parental control than Romanian girls. Grades and parental control means, by ethnic group, are shown in Table 13.1.

Interregional. A 2 (region: Banat vs. Moldova)×2 (gender) analysis of variance, with optimistic attributional style, perception of parental behaviour, grades and depressive symptoms, revealed a main effect of region on adolescents' depression, $F(1,248) = 6.40$, $p = .012$, $\eta^2 = .03$, and grades, $F(1,248) = 4.09$, $p = .044$, $\eta^2 = .07$, and a main effect of gender on grades, $F(1,248) = 15.70$, $p < .001$, $\eta^2 = .07$. Romanian

Table 13.1 Correlations between variables by ethnic/regional group (Romanians from Banat/Hungarians from Banat/Romanians from Moldova)

	M	SD	1	2	3	4
1. OAS	7.10/6.87/7.40	1.97/1.97/1.93	—	—	—	—
2. PAR	3.10/3.07/3.18	.64/.72/.76	$-.17^{\dagger}/-.38^{**}/-.29^{**}$	—	—	—
3. PCA	3.99/3.94/4.06	.69/.67/.71	$.14/.17^{\dagger}/.18^{*}$	$.001/.06/-.17^{*}$	—	—
4. CDI	10.98/11.20/13.26	6.95/5.55/8.04	$-.28^{**}/-.54^{**}/-.32^{**}$	$.37^{*}/.45^{**}/.44^{**}$	$-.18^{*}/-.20^{\dagger}/-.37^{**}$	—
5. Ach	7.71/7.88/7.41	1.46/1.54/1.36	$.26^{**}/.23^{*}/.11$	$-.22^{\dagger}/-.29^{**}/-.05$	$.28^{**}/.36^{*}/.33^{**}$	$-.22^{*}/-.35^{**}/-.20^{*}$

Romanian adolescents from Banat $N=128$, Hungarian adolescents from Banat $N=94$; Romanian adolescents from Moldova $N=127$

OAS optimistic attributional style, *PAR* parental acceptance/rejection, *PCA* parental control/autonomy, *CDI* depression, *Ach* achievement

Note: $^{**}p<.01$ level; $^{*}p<.05$; $^{\dagger}p<.09$

adolescents from Banat had a lower level of depression ($M=10.98$; SD$=6.95$) and higher grades ($M=7.71$; SD$=1.46$) than Romanian adolescents from Moldova ($M=13.26$; SD$=8.04$, $M=7.41$; SD$=1.36$, respectively). Also, Romanian girls from both regions ($M=7.88$; SD$=1.35$) had higher grades than Romanian boys ($M=7.20$; SD$=1.41$). All means, by region group, are presented in Table 13.1.

Interethnic and Interregional. A 2 (ethnicity: Romanian adolescents from Moldova vs. Hungarian adolescents from Banat)$\times$2 (gender) analysis of variance revealed main effects of ethnicity on attributional style, grades and depression, $F(1,220)=3.91, 9.37, 5.44$; $\eta^2=.01, .11, .03$, respectively; all $ps<.05$, a main effect of gender on grades and perception of parental control, $F(1,220)=20.91, 7.46$; $\eta2=.04, .11$, respectively; all $ps<.01$. Romanian adolescents from Moldova had a higher level of depression ($M=13.26$; SD$=8.04$), lower grades ($M=7.41$; SD$=1.36$) and a more optimistic attributional style ($M=7.40$; SD$=1.93$) than Hungarian adolescents ($M=11.20$; SD$=5.55$, $M=7.88$; SD$=1.54$, $M=6.87$; SD$=1.97$, respectively). Also, all girls had higher grades ($M=8.01$; SD$=1.34$) and reported a lower level of parental control ($M=4.14$; SD$=.70$) compared to boys ($M=7.22$; SD$=1.47$, $M=3.88$; SD$=.66$).

Preliminary Analyses

For all ethnic/regional groups, the results (see Table 13.1) indicated that depressive symptoms were positively associated with parental rejection and negatively with autonomy. The adolescents' grades were positively related to autonomy, and negatively to depression. For Romanian and Hungarian adolescents from Banat, the school performances were positively related to the optimistic attributional style and negatively to parental rejection.

Multiple Hierarchical Regression Predicting Students' Achievement and Depression

We computed a series of multiple regression analyses to evaluate the extent to which the effect of attributional style is mediated by parental behaviour across the samples (Aiken and West 1991). First, a series of regressions were conducted to predict students' achievement. Second, other series of regressions were conducted to predict the students' depression. In each regression, the participants' optimistic attributional style was introduced in the equation in step 1; the perceptions of parental behaviour were introduced in the equation in step 2; and the interactions between the attributional style and perceptions of parental behaviour were introduced in step 3.

The results, which are summarised in Table 13.2, showed that optimistic attributional style was a significant predictor of school performance for both Romanian ($\beta=.26, p<.01$) and Hungarian ($\beta=.26, p<.01$) adolescents from Banat, but not for the Romanian sample from Moldova ($\beta=.26$, ns). The perception of parental

Table 13.2 Hierarchical multiple regression analysis to predict school achievement

Predictors	Romanians from Banat		Hungarians from Banat		Romanians from Moldova	
	β	ΔR^2	β	ΔR^2	β	ΔR^2
Step 1						
OAS	.26**	.07**	.23*	.05*	.11	.006
	$R^2=.07, F(1,126)=9.69^{**}$		$R^2=.05, F(1,92)=5.18^{*}$		$R^2=.006, F(1,125)=1.74$	
Step 2						
PAR	−.18*	–	−.30**	–	.02	–
PCA	.25**	.09**	.37**	.18**	.33**	.10**
	$R^2=.16, F(3,124)=8.17^{**}$		$R^2=.23, F(3,90)=9.36^{**}$		$R^2=.09, F(3,126)=5.48^{**}$	
Step 3						
OAS×PAR	.14	–	.09	–	.004	–
OAS×PCA	.04	.02	−.08	.01	.03	.001
	$R^2=.18, F(5,122)=5.67^{**}$		$R^2=.25, F(5,88)=5.91^{**}$		$R^2=.08, F(5,121)=3.27^{**}$	

Romanian adolescents from Banat $N=128$, Hungarian adolescents from Banat $N=94$, Romanian adolescents from Moldova $N=127$

OAS optimistic attributional style, *PAR* parental acceptance/rejection, *PCA* parental control/autonomy

Note: $^{**}p<.01$; $^{*}p<.05$

control was a significant predictor of the achievement for Romanian and Hungarian adolescents from Banat ($\beta=.25$, $\beta=.37$, all $ps<.01$) and for Romanian adolescents from Moldova ($\beta=.33$, $p<.01$). The perception of parental acceptance was a significant predictor of achievement only for Romanian and Hungarian adolescents from Banat ($\beta=-.18$, $\beta=-30$, all $ps<.01$). The interactions between attributional style and parental behaviour were not significant.

The results, which are summarised in Table 13.3, showed that optimistic attributional style and the perception of parental behaviour were significant predictors of depression for all samples: Romanian ($\beta=-.28$, $\beta=.34$, $\beta=-.15$, all $ps<.05$) and Hungarian ($\beta=-.54$, $\beta=.30$, $\beta=-.15$, all $ps<.05$) adolescents from Banat and Romanian adolescents from Moldova ($\beta=-.32$, $\beta=.35$, $\beta=-.27$, all $ps<.01$). The interactions between attributional style and parental behaviour were not significant.

Discussion

The first goal of the present study was to examine the differences generated by ethnic/regional criteria on the adolescents' optimistic attributional style, perceptions of parental behaviour, achievement and depression. The results indicated that ethnicity had no effect on these variables. Ethnic group had a significant effect on the perception of parental control only in interaction with adolescents' gender. Our findings indicated that the regional criterion had no effect on optimistic attributional style and the perception of parental behaviour, but it influenced adolescents' depression and achievement. Romanian adolescents from Banat had a lower level of depression and higher grades than Romanian adolescents from Moldova. The predominance of similarities rather than differences on the ethnic criterion between Romanian and Hungarian students living in Banat confirms the results of previous research conducted in this region. Gavreliuc (2011) induced the idea that, in Banat, the directly shared historical experience led to the mitigation of negative interethnic attitudes so that Romanians from this region prefer to interact with their fellow citizens of other ethnicities than with the Romanians from Moldova "alike with them" as regards ethnicity.

The interregional differences found in our study, in depression and grades, may be explained through socioeconomic determinants. According to Voinea et al. (2007), Banat region has a significant higher level of social, economic and technological development than Moldova. Studies already showed that SES is critically important for achievement (Meneghan 1996; Parcel and Meneghan 1994; Pallock and Lamborn 2006). Families with a higher SES can more easily transmit cultural capital to their children, conducive to educational success, and can invest more in their children's education, while living in poverty has direct, negative effects on the cognitive ability and achievement (Bourdieu 1997; Charles et al. 2007).

Considering simultaneously ethnic and regional criteria, results highlight differences in the optimistic attributional style, except those determined only by the

Table 13.3 Hierarchical multiple regression analysis to predict depressive symptoms

Predictors	Romanians from Banat		Hungarians from Banat		Romanians from Moldova	
	B	ΔR^2	B	ΔR^2	β	ΔR^2
Step 1						
OAS	−.28**	.08**	−.54**	.29**	−.32**	.10**
	$R^2=.08, F(1,126)=10.93^{**}$		$R^2=.29, F(1,92)=39.51^{*}$		$R^2=.09, F(1,125)=14.84^{**}$	
Step 2						
PAR	.34**	–	.30**	–	.35**	–
PCA	−.16*	.13**	−.15*	.09**	−.27**	.21**
	$R^2=.19, F(3,124)=11.32^{**}$		$R^2=.37, F(3,90)=19.77^{**}$		$R^2=.30, F(3,126)=19.17^{**}$	
Step 3						
OAS×PAR	.05	–	.07	–	−.07	–
OAS×PCA	.01	.003	−.07	.009	−.11	.01
	$R^2=.19, F(5,122)=6.79^{**}$		$R^2=.37, F(5,88)=11.72^{**}$		$R^2=.30, F(5,121)=11.92^{**}$	

Romanian adolescents from Banat $N=128$, Hungarian adolescents from Banat $N=94$, Romanian adolescents from Moldova $N=127$

OAS optimistic attributional style, *PAR* parental acceptance/rejection, *PCA* parental control/autonomy

Note: $^{**}p<.01$; $^{*}p<.05$

regional factor (depression and school performance). Romanian adolescents from Moldova had a higher level of depression, lower grades, but a higher level of optimism than Hungarian adolescents from Banat. The economic, social and technological superiority of Banat region (Voinea et al. 2007) could explain the lower level of depression in this region. The surprisingly higher level in optimism of Romanians from Moldova compared to that of Hungarians from Banat could be considered as a mechanism of surviving in unfavourable conditions. The hope that tomorrow will be better helps to overcome the current difficulties. The association of high unrealistic optimism (Armor and Taylor 2002) with certain regional values, like traditions, disengagement manners, conformism and subsistence value orientations (Antohi 1997), has dysfunctional effects. This combination could determine non-involvement and could perpetuate a lower level of development in Moldova.

Our secondary aim was to examine whether there are ethnical or regional differences in the relationships between optimistic attributional style and the perception of parental behaviour, on one side, and adolescents' depression and achievement, on the other side. Our data indicated that, across all ethnic/regional groups, optimism and parental behaviour were significant predictors of depression: students who reported a more optimistic attributional style, more parental acceptance or more autonomy were more likely to report a lower level of depression. Thus, given the findings of the current study, it appears that the current hopefulness model may be applicable across ethnic and regional groups. Thus, the results confirm the assumptions of hopefulness theory (Needles and Abramson 1990). Adolescents with an optimistic attributional style had a lower level of depression than those without an optimistic attributional style. The results are consistent with other studies on adolescents (Vines and Nixon 2009; Voelz et al. 2003), which showed that optimism is a protective factor for depression (Peterson and Steen 2002).

Results confirm the relationship between parental behaviour and the adolescents' depression. Our data on parental control are convergent with previous research which demonstrated the positive association between depression and psychological control (Barber 1996; Restifo and Bögels 2009) and overcontrol (Garber et al. 1997). Also, results are in accordance with previous findings which demonstrated that parental acceptance is associated with a lower level of depression, while parental rejection and neglect is associated with a higher level of depression (An 2010; Haskett et al. 2006; Slavich et al. 2010).

The relationships between the studied variables were partially moderated by the cultural group. The relationship between achievement and both optimistic attributional style and parental acceptance was not moderated by the ethnic group. For both Romanian and Hungarian adolescents from Banat, the achievement was positively associated with optimistic attributional style and parental control. However, these relationships were not significant when considering the regional criterion. For Romanian adolescents from Moldova, the achievement level did not correlate with optimistic attributional style and parental acceptance. Our data indicated similar results in predicting the adolescents' achievement. For both Romanian and Hungarian adolescents from Banat, the optimistic attributional style and the perception of parental behaviour were significant predictors of achievement. Adolescents who reported a more optimistic attributional style, more autonomy and parental acceptance were more likely to report higher grades. Considering the regional criterion, the regression results are different. In the Romanian sample from Moldova, only parental control was a significant predictor of achievement; adolescents with more autonomy were more likely to report higher grades.

Thus, the findings of this study confirm that the optimistic attributional style had a significant impact on the adolescents' achievement; optimistic adolescents had a higher level of achievement than those without an optimistic attributional style. Due to the lack of previous research on the relationship between optimistic attributional style and achievement, it is difficult to compare the present findings to previous research. Thus, the attributional style may buffer the experience of school failure, and this idea is consistent with previous adult studies (Glasgow et al. 1997; Leeson et al. 2008). This relationship is regionally moderated; the results apply only to Romanian and Hungarian adolescents from Banat region but not to adolescents from Moldova. In the Moldova sample, the relationship between optimism and academic performance was not significant (Armor and Taylor 2002; Mezulis et al. 2004). These results may be explained through the unrealistic optimism which may determine a decrease in motivation and effort for learning activities and, consequently, a low level of achievement.

The current study had both strengths and weaknesses. A significant strength of this study lies in the simultaneous analyses of optimism on achievement and emotions of adolescent samples. Previous research analysed the relationship between optimism, achievement and depression in separate studies (Glasgow et al. 1997; Vines and Nixon 2009). Moreover, until now the relationship between optimism measured using the attributional style and adolescents' achievement was not studied. Another significant strength of this study is represented by the simultaneous analyses of ethnic and regional criteria on the relationship between optimism and adolescents' outcomes. Previous research examined if the level of optimism was determined by the regional group (Oettingen and Seligman 1990; Zullow et al. 1988). Also, the previous studies explored if the relationship between optimism and depression is mediated by ethnic group (Stein et al. 2010; Herman et al. 2007). Another significant strength of this study was the confirmation that parental acceptance and autonomy are important determinants of achievement and emotions during adolescence. Moreover, our findings suggest that variations in parental behaviour are determined by the ethnic and regional group: regional differences determined imparities in educational investment, and these inequalities persisted both across schools and across generations (Bourdieu 1997).

There were also limitations to the current study. First, the study used secondary school samples from only two towns from these regions, thus the results are not generalised to a more diverse sample. Future research needs to use an increased samples size and to include more ethnic and regional groups. A second limitation of this research relates to the disregard of the school learning environment, including the quality of instructional processes, the learning climate, the classroom goal structures, the teacher-student relationships and the student-student relationships, which may determine cognitive and affective outcomes in adolescents. Future research needs to explore more concretely the role of social network variables in the adolescents' attainment, from an ethnic and regional perspective. Third, the study used the adolescents' self-reported evaluation of parental behaviour. Even if this type of measurement is a subjective assessment of parental behaviour, it is accepted and it was used in previous studies. Using systematic behavioural observation could improve the reliability of measurement. Also, although in our study parenting practices did not moderate the relationship between optimism and adolescents' outcomes, further research is necessary to develop a clearer understanding of the development of optimistic attributional style and the manner in which its effect on adolescents' educational outcomes is moderated by parental behaviour. These results suggest that teachers may design different intervention programmes focused on adolescents' reattribution retraining, or focused on parents' retraining (to increase the adolescents' acceptance and autonomy).

In conclusion, we believe that the data bring a valuable contribution to our understanding of the role of individual and social variables in the adolescents' cognitive and affective outcomes. Although our findings may be specific to the cultural context of the study (our sample consisted of Romanian adolescents), they provide evidence for the cultural generalisation of the theoretical models. Due to the relative lack of research into social correlates of the adolescents' well-being and school outcomes in Central and Eastern Europe, we believe that the findings of the current study are particularly valuable and important for an international scientific audience. Theoretical models already explained the relationship between the studied variables, from an international and interethnic perspective, but disregarding regional particularities. This applies more in countries with regional high socioeconomic differences. The most relevant message of our study is that it highlights a less studied criterion – the regional – in analysing the relationship between the individual and social factors and the adolescents' educational outcomes.

Acknowledgement   This work was supported by CNCSIS-UEFISCDI, Project number 849 PNII_IDEI 2026/2008.

References

Abela, J. R. Z., McGirr, A., & Skitch, S. A. (2007). Depressogenic inferential styles, negative events, and depressive symptoms in youth: An attempt to reconcile past inconsistent findings. *Behaviour Research and Therapy, 45,* 2397–2406.

Abramson, L. J., Seligman, M. E. P., & Teasdale, J. D. (1978). Learned helplessness in humans: Critique and reformulation. *Journal of Abnormal Psychology, 87,* 49–74.

Abramson, L. Y., Metalsky, G. I., & Alloy, B. (1989). Hopelessness depression: A theory-based subtype of depression. *Psychological Review, 96*(2), 358–372.

Aiken, L. S., & West, S. G. (1991). *Multiple regression: Testing and interpreting interactions.* Newburg Park: Sage.

An, B. P. (2010). The relations between race, family characteristics, and where students apply to college. *Social Science Research, 39,* 310–323.

Antohi, S. (1997). *Exercise of distance* [Exercițiul distanței]. București: Nemira.

Armor, D. A., & Taylor, S. E. (2002). When predictions fail: The dilemma of unrealistic optimism. In T. Gilovich, D. Griffin, & D. Kahneman (Eds.), *Heuristics and biases: The psychology of intuitive judgment* (pp. 334–347). Cambridge: Cambridge University Press.

Barber, B. K. (1996). Parental psychological control: Revisiting a neglected construct. *Child Development, 67*, 2396–3319.

Baumrind, D. (1991). Parenting styles and adolescent development. In J. Brooks-Gunn, R. Lerner, & A. C. Petersen (Eds.), *The encyclopedia of adolescence* (pp. 746–758). New York: Garland.

Bernardo, A. B. I. (2010). Exploring Filipino adolescents' perceptions of the legitimacy of parental authority over academic behaviors. *Journal of Applied Developmental Psychology, 31*, 273–280.

Bodovski, K., & Youn, M. J. (2010). Love, discipline and elementary school achievement: The role of family emotional climate. *Social Science Research, 39*, 585–595.

Bourdieu, P. (1997). Cultural reproduction and social reproduction. In J. Karabel & A. H. Halsey (Eds.), *Power and ideology in education* (pp. 487–511). New York: Oxford University Press.

Bradley, R. H., & Corwyn, R. F. (2004). "Family process" investments that matter for child well being. In A. Kalil & T. Delayer (Eds.), *Family investment in children's potential* (pp. 1–32). Mahwah: Erlbaum.

Bronfenbrenner, U. (1979). *The ecology of human development.* Cambridge, MA: Harvard University Press.

Bronfenbrenner, U., & Morris, P. A. (1998). Theoretical models of human development. In W. Damon & R. M. Lerner (Eds.), *Handbook of child psychology* (Vol. 1, pp. 993–1028). New York: Wiley.

Butnaru, S., Gherasim, L. R., Iacob, L., & Amariei, C. (2010). The effects of parental support and attributional style on children's school achievement and depressive feelings. *The International Journal of Learning, 17*(8), 397–408.

Charles, C. Z., Roscigno, V. J., & Torres, K. C. (2007). Racial inequality and college attendance: The mediating role of parental investments. *Social Science Research, 36*, 329–352.

Cheng, H., & Furnham, A. (2003). Attributional style and self-esteem as predictors of psychological well being. *Counseling Psychology Quarterly, 16*(2), 121–130.

Ciarrochi, J., Heaven, P. C. L., & Davies, F. (2007). The impact of hope, self-esteem, and attributional style on adolescents' school grades and emotional well-being: A longitudinal study. *Journal of Research in Personality, 41*, 1161–1178.

Conley, C. S., Haines, B. A., Hilt, L. M., & Metalsky, G. I. (2001). The children's attributional style interview: Developmental tests of cognitive diathesis-stress theories of depression. *Journal of Abnormal Child Psychology, 29*, 445–463.

Curry, J., & Craighead, W. (1990). Attributional style in clinically depressed and conduct disordered adolescents. *Journal of Consulting and Clinical Psychology, 58*, 109–115.

Fresco, D. M., Alloy, L. B., & Reilly-Harrington, N. (2006). Association of attributional style for negative and positive events and the occurrence of life events with depression and anxiety. *Journal of Social and Clinical Psychology, 25*, 1140–1159.

Garber, J., Robinson, N. S., & Valentiner, D. (1997). The relation between parenting and adolescent depression: Self-worth as a mediator. *Journal of Adolescent Research, 12*, 12–33.

Gavreliuc, A. (2011). *Romanias from Romania. Autarchic individualism, transgenerational value patterns and social autism* [Româniile din România. Individualism autarhic, tipare valorice transgeneraționale și autism social]. Timișoara: Editura Universității de Vest.

Glasgow, K., Dornbusch, S., Troyer, L., Steinberg, L., & Ritter, P. (1997). Parenting styles, adolescents' attributions, and educational outcomes in nine heterogeneous high schools. *Child Development, 68*, 507–529.

Greaven, S. H., Santor, D. A., Thompson, R., & Zuroff, D. C. (2000). Adolescent self-handicapping, depressive affect, and maternal parenting styles. *Journal of Youth and Adolescence, 29*, 631–646.

Haeffel, G. J., & Vargas, I. (2011). Resilience to depressive symptoms: The buffering effects of enhancing cognitive style and positive life events. *Journal of Behavior Therapy and Experimental Psychiatry, 42*, 13–18.

Harwood, R. L. (1992). The influence of culturally derived values on Anglo and Puerto Rican mothers' perceptions of attachment behavior. *Child Development, 63*, 822–839.

Haskett, M. E., Nears, K., Sabourin Ward, C., & McPherson, A. V. (2006). Diversity in adjustment of maltreated children: Factors associated with resilient functioning. *Clinical Psychology Review, 26*(6), 796–812.

Herman, K. C., Ostrander, R., & Tucker, C. M. (2007). Do family environments and negative cognitions of adolescents with depressive symptoms vary by ethnic group? *Journal of Family Psychology, 21*, 325–330.

Hipwell, A., Keenan, K., Kasza, K., Loeber, R., Stouthamer-Loeber, M., & Bean, T. (2008). Reciprocal influences between girls' conduct problems and depression, and parental punishment and warmth: A six year prospective analysis. *Journal of Abnormal Child Psychology, 36*(5), 663–677.

Hughes, D. L., & Seidman, E. (2002). In pursuit of a culturally anchored methodology. In T. A. Revenson, A. R. D'Augelli, S. E. French, D. L. Hughes, D. Livert, E. Seidman, M. Shinn, & H. Yoshikawa (Eds.), *Ecological research to promote social change: Methodological advances from community psychology* (pp. 243–255). New York: Kluwer Academic/Plenum Publishers.

Johnson, J. G., Han, Y. S., Douglas, C. J., Johannet, C. M., & Russell, T. (1998). Attributions for positive life events predict recovery from depression among psychiatric inpatients: An investigation of the Needles and Abramson model of recovery from depression. *Journal of Counseling and Clinical Psychology, 66*(2), 369–376.

Juang, L. P., Syed, M., & Takagi, M. (2007). Intergenerational discrepancies of parental control among Chinese American families: Links to family conflict and adolescent depressive symptoms. *Journal of Adolescence, 30*, 965–975.

Kovacs, M. (1985). The children's depression inventory (CDI). *Psychopharmacology Bulletin, 21*, 995–998.

Leeson, P., Ciarrochi, J., & Heaven, P. C. L. (2008). Cognitive ability, personality, and academic performance in adolescence. *Personality and Individual Differences, 45*, 630–635.

Lieber, E., Yang, K., & Lin, Y. (2000). An external orientation to the study of causal beliefs: Applications to Chinese populations and comparative research. *Journal of Cross-Cultural Psychology, 31*, 160–186.

Mahtani, M., Kennard, B. D., Hughes, C. W., Mayes, T. L., Emslie, G. J., Lee, P. W., & Lewinshon, P. M. (2004). A cross-cultural investigation and depressive symptoms in adolescents. *Journal of Abnormal Psychology, 113*(2), 248–257.

Martin-Krumm, C. P., Sarrazin, P. G., & Peterson, C. (2005). The moderating effects of explanatory style in physical education performance: A prospective study. *Personality and Individual Differences, 38*, 1645–1656.

Meneghan, E. G. (1996). Family composition, family interaction, and children's academic and behavior problems: Interpreting the data. In A. Booth & J. F. Dunn (Eds.), *Family-school links: How do they affect educational outcomes?* (pp. 185–196). Mahwah: Lawrence Erlbaum.

Mezulis, A. H., Abramson, L. Y., Hyde, J. S., & Hankin, B. L. (2004). Is there a universal positivity bias in attributions: A meta-analytic review of individual, developmental, and cultural differences in the self-serving attributional bias. *Psychological Bulletin, 130*(5), 711–747.

Michiels, D., Grietens, H., Onghena, P., & Kuppens, S. (2008). Parent-child interactions and relational aggression in peer relationships. *Developmental Review, 28*, 522–540.

Morris, M. C., Ciesla, J. A., & Garber, J. (2008). A prospective study of the cognitive-stress model of depressive symptoms in adolescents. *Journal of Abnormal Psychology, 117*(4), 719–734.

Needles, D. J., & Abramson, L. Y. (1990). Positive life events, attributional style, and hopefulness: Testing a model of recovery from depression. *Journal of Abnormal Psychology, 99*(2), 156–165.

Nsamenang, A. B., & Lamb, M. E. (1994). Socialization of Nso children in the Bamende Grassfields of Northwest Cameroon. In P. M. Greenfield & R. R. Cocking (Eds.), *Cross-cultural roots of minority child development* (pp. 133–146). Hillsdale: Lawrence Erlbaum Associates Publishers.

Oettingen, G., & Seligman, M. E. P. (1990). Pessimism and behavioral signs of depression in East versus West Berlin. *European Journal of Social Psychology, 20,* 207–220.

Openshaw, D. K., Darwin, L. T., & Rollins, B. C. (1984). Parental influences of adolescent self-esteem. *The Journal of Early Adolescence, 4,* 259–263.

Pallock, L. L., & Lamborn, S. D. (2006). Beyond parenting practices: Extended kinship support and the academic adjustment of African-American and European-American teens. *Journal of Adolescence, 29,* 813–828.

Parcel, T., & Meneghan, E. G. (1994). *Parents' jobs and children's lives.* New York: Aldine de Gruyter.

Peterson, C., & Seligman, M. E. P. (1984). Causal explanations as a risk factor for depression: Theory and evidence. *Psychological Review, 91,* 347–374.

Peterson, C., & Steen, T. A. (2002). Optimistic explanatory style. In C. R. Snyder & S. J. Lopez (Eds.), *Handbook of positive psychology* (pp. 244–256). Oxford: Oxford University Press.

Repinski, D. J., & Shonk, S. M. (2002). Mothers' and fathers' behavior, adolescents' self-representations and adolescents' adjustment: A mediational model. *The Journal of Early Adolescence, 22,* 357–368.

Restifo, K., & Bögels, S. M. (2009). Family processes in the development of youth depression: Translating the evidence to treatment. *Clinical Psychology Review, 29,* 294–316.

Richman, A. L., Miller, P. M., & Solomon, M. J. (1988). The socialization of infants in suburban Boston. In R. A. LeVine, P. M. Miller, & M. M. West (Eds.), *New directions for child development: Parental behavior in diverse societies* (Vol. 40, pp. 65–74). San Francisco: Jossey-Bass.

Rothon, C., Head, J., Klineberg, E., & Stansfeld, S. (2011). Can social support protect adolescents from adverse outcomes? A prospective study on the effects of bullying on the educational achievement and mental health of adolescents at secondary schools in East London. *Journal of Adolescence, 34,* 579–588.

Sandu, D. (2003). *Sociability in the space of development. Trust, tolerance and social networks* [Sociabilitatea în spaţiul dezvoltării. Încredere, toleranţă şi reţele sociale]. Iaşi: Polirom.

Sanjuan, P., & Magallares, A. (2009). A longitudinal study of the negative explanatory style and attributions of uncontrollability as predictors of depressive symptoms. *Personality and Individual Differences, 46,* 714–718.

Schaefer, E. S. (1965). Children's report of parental behavior: An inventory. *Child Development, 36,* 413–424.

Scheier, M. F., & Carver, C. S. (1985). Optimism, coping, and health: Assessment and implication of generalized outcome expectancies. *Health Psychology, 4,* 219–247.

Schludermann, E., & Schludermann, S. (1970). Replicability of factors in children's report of parent behavior. *Journal of Psychology, 76,* 239–249.

Slavich, G. M., O'Donovan, A., Epel, E. S., & Kemeny, M. E. (2010). Black sheep get the blues: A psychobiological model of social rejection and depression. *Neuroscience and Biobehavioral Reviews, 35,* 39–45.

Soenens, B., & Vansteenkiste, M. (2010). A theoretical upgrade of the concept of parental psychological control: Proposing new insights on the basis of self-determination theory. *Developmental Review, 30,* 74–99.

Stein, G. L., Curry, J. F., Hersh, J., Breland-Noble, A., March, J., Silva, S. D., Reinecke, M. A., & Jacobs, R. (2010). Ethnic differences among adolescents beginning treatment for depression. *Cultural Diversity and Ethnic Minority Psychology, 16*(2), 152–158.

Thompson, M., Kaslow, N. J., Weiss, B., & Nolan-Hoeksema, S. (1998). Children's attributional style questionnaire–revised: Psychometric examination. *Psychological Assessment, 10,* 166–170.

Triandis, H. C. (2001). Individualism-collectivism and personality. *Journal of Personality, 69,* 907–924.

Vines, L., & Nixon, R. D. V. (2009). Positive attributional style, life events and their effect on children's mood: Prospective study. *Australian Journal of Psychology, 61*(4), 211–219.

Voelz, Z., Haeffel, G., Joiner, T., & Wagner, K. (2003). Reducing hopelessness: The interaction of enhancing and depressogenic attributional styles for positive and negative life events among youth psychiatric inpatients. *Behavior Research and Therapy, 41*, 1183–1198.

Voicu, B., & Voicu, M. (2007). *Romanians' values: 1993–2006. A sociological perspective* [Valori ale românilor: 1993–2006. O perspectivă sociologică]. Iaşi: Editura Institutul European.

Voinea, L., Cojanu, V., Lungu, L., Sandu, D., & Şerb, I. (2007). *Romania – Building regional assessment capacity in line with the Lisbon agenda* (pp. 42–46). Bucharest: British Embassy.

Watkins, D., Mortazavi, S., & Trofimova, I. (2000). Independent and interdependent conceptions of self: An investigation of age, gender, and culture differences in important and satisfaction ratings. *Cross Cultural Research, 34*, 113–134.

Yang, S., & Shin, C. S. (2008). Parental attitudes towards education: What matters for children's well-being? *Children and Youth Services Review, 30*, 1328–1335.

Yates, S. M., & Yates, G. C. R. (1995). Explanatory style, ego-orientation and primary school mathematics. *Educational Psychology, 15*, 28–34.

Zullow, H. M., Oettingen, G., Peterson, C., & Seligman, M. E. P. (1988). Pessimistic explanatory style in the historical record. *American Psychologist, 43*(9), 673–682.

Index

H.H. Knoop and A. Delle Fave (eds.), *Well-Being and Cultures: Perspectives
from Positive Psychology*, Cross-Cultural Advancements in Positive Psychology 3,
DOI 10.1007/978-94-007-4611-4, © Springer Science+Business Media Dordrecht 2013